"If I had to sum up this book in one word, the word would be 'brilliant'! This is one of the most insightful books on TOC, not just for healthcare, that I have ever read."
—Bob Sproull, author of *The Ultimate Improvement Cycle: Maximizing Profits through the Integration of Lean, Six Sigma, and the Theory of Constraints*

"As a physician practicing in a managed care environment, I do face and deal with the increasing complexity and dysfunction of the healthcare system. We, the physicians, struggle to provide best possible care for our patients; however, the institutions lack the tools to identify and eliminate the root causes preventing the system from achieving better global outcomes. *Performance Improvement for Healthcare* is a practical guided process to direct efforts at the point of leverage for sustained improvement."
—Seza Gulec, MD, FACS
Professor of Surgery and
Radiology/Nuclear Medicine

"Less variation, less waste, and no patient safety issues, together with better medical and financial outcomes, higher efficiency, and patient satisfaction—I think that all this is possible. This book shows the direction."
—Metin Çakmakçi, MD, MS, FACS, FACPE
Professor of Surgery
Medical Director, ASM

Performance Improvement for Healthcare

Leading Change with Lean, Six Sigma, and Constraints Management

Bahadir Inozu, Ph.D.

Dan Chauncey, MA, MBA, LSSMBB

Vickie Kamataris, RN, CPHQ, LSSMBB

Charles Mount, CAPT, NC, USN, RN, M.Ed.

NOVACES, LLC

New York   Chicago   San Francisco
Lisbon   London   Madrid   Mexico City
Milan   New Delhi   San Juan
Seoul   Singapore   Sydney   Toronto

McGraw-Hill books are available at special quantity discounts to use as premiums and sales promotions, or for use in corporate training programs. To contact a representative, please e-mail us at bulksales@mcgraw-hill.com.

Performance Improvement for Healthcare:
Leading Change with Lean, Six Sigma, and Constraints Management

1 2 3 4 5 6 7 8 9 0   DOC/DOC   1 7 6 5 4 3 2 1

ISBN   978-0-07-176162-8
MHID   0-07-176162-4

The pages within this book were printed on acid-free paper.

Sponsoring Editor
Judy Bass

Editorial Supervisor
Stephen M. Smith

Production Supervisor
Richard C. Ruzycka

Project Manager
Patricia Wallenburg, TypeWriting

Copy Editor
James Madru

Proofreader
Claire Splan

Indexer
Claire Splan

Art Director, Cover
Jeff Weeks

Composition
TypeWriting

From Baha: To my loving parents, Ayşe Berruh and Mehmet Oğuz İnözü.

From Dan: To my wife, Wanda, for understanding all the time away making this (both the book and the work we are doing in healthcare) happen.

From Vickie: To my family for their love and support and sacrifice, their understanding and acceptance of my need to care for others. To God for the capacity to do so.

From Charles: To my wife, Irene, family and friends for their tremendous support, guidance and encouragement.

About the Authors

Bahadir Inozu, Ph.D., is a Founding Partner and the Chief Executive Officer of NOVACES, a leading provider of continuous process improvement and project management consulting and training services. He is a Lean Six Sigma Master Black Belt and a Theory of Constraints Jonah. Dr. Inozu has more than 20 years of performance-improvement experience in government and the healthcare, maritime, and maintenance, repair, and overhaul (MRO) industries. He led more than 20 major applied research projects and wrote more than 70 journal articles and conference papers while he was a professor at the University of New Orleans.

Dan Chauncey, MA, MBA, LSSMBB, is the Director of Deployment Services for NOVACES, where he has served as the technical program manager for the deployment of CPI over patient care in the U.S. Navy Medical Enterprise. He also leads a team of five Master Black Belts embedded at mid-level commands across the U.S. Navy and led the CPI deployment at United Health Services.

Vickie Kamataris, RN, CPHQ, LSSMBB, is the Director of Commercial Healthcare Services for NOVACES. She is a Lean Six Sigma Master Black Belt and a registered nurse with multiple certifications, including CPHQ. In her role as Quality Leader for General Electric's Corporate Healthcare and Medical Program and as a NOVACES consultant, she has extensive experience leading interdisciplinary, global teams to achieve extraordinary improvements in a broad range of clinical and business processes.

Charles Mount, CAPT, NC, USN, RN, M.Ed., is the Director of Government Healthcare Services for NOVACES, and an ASQ-certified Lean Six Sigma Black Belt. He oversees Lean Six Sigma and Leadership programs to improve patient care, safety, and satisfaction. Captain Mount was Commanding Officer and Executive Officer of the Naval Schools of Health Sciences Training in Portsmouth, Virginia, and San Diego, California, where he coordinated the implementation of Total Quality Management for 5,000 employees.

CONTENTS

FOREWORD

This book is a survival manual. It's as simple as that.

As a retired surgeon and healthcare system CEO, I look at the challenges facing today's healthcare executives and wonder how they can possibly prevail against them.

In a recent article in *Becker's Hospital Review*, author Leigh Page clearly articulates the formidable problems that must be confronted. These include lower reimbursements, decreased state Medicaid funding, increased uncompensated care, Medicare recovery audits, and uncertainty about the impact of the Health Care Reform Act.

If these were not enough, add the daily frustrations facing healthcare providers and those who support them. They see the inefficiencies, unnecessary redundancies, and constant rework. They see the need for change but have no idea what that change should look like.

My thought is this: If Jack Welch (General Electric) and Bob Galvin (Motorola) can turn their companies around, then the bright, enterprising physicians, nurses, and administrative leaders of our healthcare organizations can do the same. But to do so, they will need the most robust methodologies and the most mature, time-tested tools. Welcome to *Performance Improvement for Healthcare: Leading Change with Lean, Six Sigma, and Constraints Management*.

For the first time, there is a fully-integrated performance improvement system that combines Constraints Management, Lean, and Six Sigma. Their synergies are powerful and dynamic and solve tough problems. Written in the language of healthcare, *Performance Improvement for Healthcare* features numerous concrete, relevant, real-life examples of successful applications of this performance-improvement system in hospital and clinic settings. It is readable, understandable, and implementable.

Leading the organizational and cultural transformation to implement these methodologies is not easy. It takes commitment, dedication, and constancy of purpose. It also requires a high degree of trust, especially among physicians, nurses, and their executive counterparts and between managers and those who report to them. However, it is doable—in fact, it's already being done.

Performance Improvement for Healthcare shows a pathway to the future of healthcare. Enjoy this book—enjoy the rewarding journey.

Robert B. Halder, MD
Rear Admiral, U.S. Navy (Ret.)

PREFACE

On November 16, 1960, at 3:00 A.M., I was being strangled by my umbilical cord. A doctor asked how my mother was feeling. She explained that she was feeling better after some minor discomfort she had been experiencing. Fortunately, the doctor decided to check my fetal heartbeat in utero just in case. The doctor determined that my heartbeat was extremely slow and that I was about to die. The doctor rushed my mother to the operating room for an emergency cesarean section. My life was saved. I am thankful that the system worked in this instance. Many other babies have not been as fortunate. In fact, witnessing the preventable deaths of two babies was so painful that it triggered a career change and a passion to improve healthcare processes and systems for one of this book's coauthors.

Fast forward 20 years: I was an intern in the engine room of a commercial cargo ship in the summer of 1980. In a three-month period, almost every piece of equipment had failed in that engine room. We even had a major fire. I felt that there had to be a better way to maintain ships such as mine to at least diminish the seemingly never-ending failures. That experience brought me to the University of Michigan to better understand reliability and maintenance of ship machinery and how to improve them.

Then, at a maintenance conference, I heard about Six Sigma, which was developed by a reliability engineer. After studying it further and implementing it to improve the availability of shipyard cranes, I realized the power of Six Sigma. Yes, I was aware of most of its tools before. However, using those tools within the discipline of the Six Sigma roadmap, combined with the soft skills of change management and project management, brought much more powerful, sustainable results. This was when Lean, Six Sigma, and Constraints Management were like competing professional sports teams where each practitioner believed that his or her method was the best.

Then I saw a trend to integrate Lean and Six Sigma. A growing number of practitioners recognized that the methodologies were complementary. The U.S. Navy provided a research grant to my team at the University of New Orleans to pioneer Lean Six Sigma integration in shipbuilding at

Northrop Grumman Ship Systems. The success of that project gave birth to NOVACES, which was founded by the project's researchers. Next, we were invited to the core contractor team to truly integrate Constraints Management with Lean Six Sigma in the largest supply-chain network in the world: the U.S. Naval Aviation Enterprise. The synergy between the methodologies was even more apparent than the differences. Subsequently, we had the opportunity to adopt and apply the integrated approach first to Navy hospitals and clinics and then to other health systems worldwide. Our passion to improve healthcare performance brought us together to write this book. Our diverse backgrounds allowed us to bring the latest methodologies to healthcare from various perspectives. In this journey, my path first crossed that of coauthor Dan Chauncey. Here is his story:

After more than 10 years in law enforcement, I found myself serving as a trainer and quality-assurance leader for the U.S. Air Force Corrections Facility in Denver, Colorado. In this role, I had the opportunity to have my position audited by the local personnel office. I was absolutely astonished to find that the auditor assessed that all the effort I put into my long workdays was worth only *one-half* of a full-time equivalent (FTE). I immediately balked at this finding and asked for help in understanding how such a conclusion was reached. I was amazed that once I understood the rules and operational definitions, I could not refute the findings. I was so intrigued that I made the decision to change careers and transferred to the Air Force Management Engineering Agency to work on performance improvement and staffing analysis.

After attending the Air Force training course in Biloxi, Mississippi, I relocated to Albuquerque, New Mexico, to work within the Air Force security and law enforcement community. One of the things I realized was that the approach being applied required 26 months to complete and not a single one had been approved and implemented in three years. In my first meeting with my new commanding officer, I asked why we even bother when we get results such as these. Luckily, he had an open mind and asked if I had a solution. I stated that I "would get some smart cops (subject-matter experts) in a room and figure out how to improve the way the work was done and then cost it out." At the time, I viewed this as *common sense* and knew virtually nothing about facilitation and teams. After the commanding officer told me to "run with it," I started learning about facilitation and teams—quickly!

The first project I lead thereafter was completed within 13 months. Not only was it completed in half the time of the average project, but it also actually was approved and implemented immediately and even resulted in significant savings. The project's success led to my transfer to San Antonio, Texas, to document and standardize the approach across the Air Force. After publishing the *Air Force Regulation*, I was directed to develop a curriculum and begin training practitioners across the Air Force management engineering community. I ran the training program for around two years, and then I was assigned to be the quality advisor to the Air Force Management Engineering Agency leadership team. This was when Total Quality Management was emerging within the Air Force. It was at an extensive training program at the Air Force Quality Institute (which since has been disbanded) that I was first *really* exposed to the quality profession.

My next career transition was to spend three years as the manager of management engineering for the claims-processing center of the health insurance agency Humana. This experience gave me an opportunity to hone some data-analysis skills in a healthcare setting. After Humana, I moved to the University Health System as a quality trainer. My role was to develop training for all employees on the systems approach to process improvement. After 18 months of training delivery, it became apparent to me that training was not enough and that my team was not receiving any return on the investment. I submitted a plan to change course and was promoted to a newly developed position of Director of Performance Improvement and Organizational Development. My plan included the deployment of Six Sigma throughout the system and my attendance of Black Belt training. However, it quickly became apparent that a proper deployment of Six Sigma did not have the leadership support that was necessary for it to succeed.

I decided to move into consulting, where I reasoned that there would be more support of leadership. Since consultants are hired for the explicit purpose of improving client organizations, implicit in my role would be the vested support of the managers who brought me in and wanted a change from the status quo. I wound up working at Rath and Strong, the oldest continuously operating management consulting firm in the United States. I began working with a team of Master Black Belts deploying Six Sigma— later expanding to include Lean—to Fortune 500 companies. What a growth opportunity for me. I was exposed to virtually every industry, working with such companies as Johnson & Johnson, Pfizer, Alstom, Schneider Electric, and Aon not only in the United States but also in France, Great Britain, and Bermuda. It was this role, along with my healthcare experience, that brought me to NOVACES.

At NOVACES, I was exposed to Constraints Management and began to understand that the best way to drive improvement was to apply the right tool at the right time to the right problem—but always from a systems perspective. The natural extension of this principle was the development of SystemCPI and the integrated approach to performance improvement. When I look back at my *younger days*, I believe that my time in law enforcement, where I was trained to handle challenging situations and people—including certification as a hostage negotiator—balanced with my time in management engineering—learning the math—has positioned me well for my current role. Even my education—a master of arts in resource development and a master of business administration—contributed to a balance between *hard* and *soft skills;* a firm grasp of the balance between costs and benefits, theory and reality, and data and people; and a strong grounding in real-world practicality. Now I go to work every day (luckily some days it is right down the hall to my home office) knowing that I can contribute to making a difference in the delivery of healthcare not only in the United States but across the world.

When Dan joined NOVACES in 2006, he was passionate about Six Sigma—he still is, but he greatly appreciates its synergies with other methodologies. During the course of writing this book, we had lively debates about how to best integrate Constraints Management with Lean, Six Sigma, and other points of view to provide the best value for performance improvement in healthcare. Working on both the hospital and insurance sides of the system has given him a unique perspective and an ability to understand the highly complex relationship among people and processes in healthcare. Along the way, in 2007, Vickie Kamataris joined us. Here is her story:

I became a nurse because I wanted to make a difference. In early 1996, I was working as the patient care coordinator in a large family birth center in a large Midwestern city. My staff was well trained, disciplined, and dedicated. I ran a "tight ship" and was constantly benchmarking and seeking ways to improve performance and service to our customers. Still, bad things happened despite the best people working extraordinarily hard. Two bad outcomes occurred within a short period of time. In both cases, no one was to blame. Procedure was followed. No one did anything wrong. Still, two babies died, and I was stunned.

During this time, my husband was coming home from work every day complaining about the "latest, next best thing" at General Electric. At that time, he was manager of one of GE's major aircraft engine lines. I will never forget looking over his shoulder and reading the binder he had laid out on the table. Still, even after so many years, I get goose bumps. I *knew* that Six Sigma could change the world. My world! I determined right then to find a way to get my hands on this methodology and apply it to healthcare processes.

I resigned from the hospital and took a position at GE as an independently contracted occupational health nurse. My objective was to learn as much about Six Sigma as possible. As a contractor, I was not eligible for training. So I watched and learned, asked questions, . . . and waited. When, six months later the human resources manager came to me and asked what it would take for me to accept a GE position as the site occupational health and safety manager, my response did not surprise him. He laughed when I said, "Six Sigma training!" I was enrolled in the next wave of Green Belt training. My objective was to become certified as a Green Belt and return to the hospital with this powerful new tool.

This was early in GE's Six Sigma deployment. It was the second wave of Green Belts trained at the site. All my fellow students were managers and engineers. My Black Belt trainers were engineers. Everyone (except me) agreed that Six Sigma did not apply to transactional processes and certainly not to health and safety. It was agreed that I would need to complete a "real" training project in addition to the one I had submitted for approval. My certification project was intended to reduce the cost of handling scrap parts from one of the engine lines. The objective of my pet project was to reduce the incidence of upper extremity repetitive-stress injuries (RSI) in a rework shop.

I knew that the rework shop had a high incidence of upper extremity RSI because I had treated these injuries in the clinic, managed the medical care and disability of those who suffered from them, and reported the cost associated with lost work days and worker's compensation. I knew that the company had invested in every conceivable ergonomic improvement, including vacuum lift devices, vibration-dampened tools, and ergonomically designed tables and chairs. I had implemented exercise and nutritional programs. Still, the incidence of RSI continued to increase in this one area of the facility. I did not believe that it was a function of demographics alone (mostly women over age 50).

The engine scrap project was a success. I learned to use the tools and improved the process, saving a modest amount of money. The RSI project identified a previously unsuspected cause for RSI, and once it was corrected, the incidence of new cases and aggravation of existing cases decreased dramatically, with savings estimated at more than $170,000 per year. Soon after the project was entered into the company database, I was contacted by the medical director of GE's Corporate Healthcare and Medical Programs and invited to showcase my project at the annual medical conference in Toronto. The project was recognized as an innovation (the first healthcare-related project at GE) and a best practice (using Six Sigma to solve a clinical problem). In September, I was invited to join the corporate team in Fairfield as a project leader. I would create a balanced scorecard for GE's global network of more than 200 occupational health clinics and lead nurses and physicians to use Six Sigma to improve compliance, quality, and patient satisfaction while reducing costs.

My professional vision was to translate Six Sigma and balanced scorecard and, later, other quality tools and methods for application to healthcare processes and problems. I led clinical teams to improve performance and meet corporate objectives. I was certified as a Black Belt and then a Master Black Belt and promoted to quality leader for corporate healthcare and medical programs. In this role, I had the opportunity to present at national and international conferences, teaching nurses and other healthcare professionals beyond GE what I had learned. I created tools and templates for healthcare, including a "Define-Measure-Analyze-Improve-Control (DMAIC) in a Box" that would allow contracted nurses to improve performance without formal training. Constantly researching emerging trends and tools, I was inspired by the work being done at Virginia Mason to add Lean to my toolset well before the method was accepted by the company at large. Healthcare was beginning to see the light! In 2007, I saw my advancing career at GE evolving farther and farther away from clinical healthcare. Nursing is not what I do—it's *who I am.* The time had come for me to take the skills and knowledge I had acquired back to the hospital and clinic, pharmacy, and lab. The means by which to do this in the broadest possible sense was as a consultant.

As a NOVACES consultant, I have had the opportunity to learn from colleagues with varied backgrounds and areas of expertise to use

Constraints Management, TRIZ (which is a Russian acronym for *Teoriya Resheniya Izobretatelskikh Zadatch*, commonly known as the *Theory of Inventive Problem Solving*), and other methods to solve healthcare problems in innovative and unusual ways. I have led performance-improvement teams in military and civilian hospitals and health systems in the United States and abroad. I have trained and mentored healthcare practitioners from cooks to surgeons and touched virtually every healthcare process. I have had the opportunity to lead deployments, projects, and events from the Bureau of Medicine in Washington, DC, to Anadolu in Gebze, Turkey. I am able . . . every day . . . to *make a difference.*

And Vickie indeed makes a *big* difference with her passion, dedication, and unwillingness to rest on her laurels. Even after she was a pioneer, applying Six Sigma to healthcare when even GE did not believe it could be done, she continues to have the courage to try new tools and push the methodology farther than it has ever gone before. She was convinced to join the Healthcare Division of NOVACES because it allowed her an unparalleled opportunity to achieve *real* clinical and organizational improvements for patients. Today, Vickie works closely with Charles Mount, a veteran of not only the U.S. Navy but also of quality improvement in healthcare. Here is his story:

While stationed at the Naval School of Health Sciences in Bethesda, Maryland, I had an outstanding opportunity to teach the Navy Medicine's leadership and management education and training (LMET) curriculum for midlevel healthcare professionals in Navy hospitals throughout the nation. It was a two-week, competency-based course taught on the road at the hospitals and medical centers, training newly promoted department heads, division officers, and special assistants in how to lead and manage highly skilled experts effectively in healthcare. During a coffee break, my boss, a senior Navy captain, rushed upstairs and yelled, "Charles, we need a TQM [Total Quality Management] bibliography on Dr. Deming's work for the senior class, and we need it now!"

While I had heard about TQM and W. Edwards Deming, at that time, I had only peripheral knowledge of his work. I asked the captain where he thought I should start. He quickly replied, "Call his office at George Washington University and see if you can talk with him." I called George Washington University and was unable to actually talk with Dr. Deming, but I did talk with his administrative assistant, who sent me his bibliography. Little did I realize the extraordinary journey I had embarked on in process improvement.

At the time, the Navy used the term *Total Quality Management* (TQM) synonymously with *Continuous Process Improvement*. (The Chief of Naval Operations later changed it to *Total Quality Leadership* to highlight the Navy's emphasis on leadership rather than management.) On transfer to the Naval Medical Center in San Diego (NMCSD), the Navy's largest healthcare system, I was appointed as the special assistant for TQM to the commanding officer, Rear Admiral Robert Halder. Dr. Halder was a highly respected admiral, physician, and leader throughout the Navy. My first goal at Dr. Halder's command was to learn as much as I could about Continuous Process Improvement (CPI) and to do so as quickly as possible. The admiral believed in the immersion style of learning and sent me to six TQL-CPI courses in seven weeks. I was literally *drenched* in all the tools, methods, concepts, and skills of CPI, including the Hospital Corporation of America's model of find-organize-clarify-understand-select (FOCUS)–plan-do-check-act (PDCA).

Dr. Halder fully understood the power of CPI, having just returned from attending the Navy Surgeon General's conference on CPI for all his admirals. During that conference, the audience heard a presentation by Dr. Donald Berwick regarding National Demonstration Project (NDP) efforts to implement the industrial tools of TQM in healthcare. What Dr. Halder heard resonated with his style of medical practice. Additionally, he believed wholeheartedly in the top-down approach at NMCSD and wanted to accelerate the implementation of TQM himself. In order to accomplish this effectively, he asked me to quickly meet with San Diego area hospitals and create a coalition with which he could then bring Dr. Berwick's presentation to San Diego. I met with the performance-improvement coordinators at two large medical centers and created the Southern California Coalition for Improving Healthcare Quality.

I served as president of the Southern California Coalition for Improving Healthcare Quality for six years. At its peak, 24 hospitals from San Diego and Orange County attended its meetings and conferences. The coalition sponsored numerous healthcare conferences and workshops, all with one primary intent: to help the hospitals and their medical, nursing, administrative, and allied staff implement the principles and practices of CPI. Thus the coalition became a support group, a mentoring team, and an accelerator for healthcare's deployment of CPI throughout San Diego.

Coincidentally, on my arrival in San Diego, I was introduced to the San Diego Deming User Group (DUG). The group had been started by Dr. Deming himself when he was asked to assist the North Island Naval Rework Facility, which repaired the engines on the Navy's fighter jets. Dr. Deming contributed his own money to create the group and conducted the first meetings.

Starting as the education director, I later became vice president and then president of this group. The DUG also sponsored numerous CPI training programs and conferences and enabled many members to attend Dr. Deming's famous four-day conferences. With the combination of the coalition and the DUG, San Diego's healthcare system quickly embraced CPI and saw a remarkable impact on its hospitals' delivery of healthcare. At NMCSD, the results included over 50 process action teams and savings well into the millions of dollars.

As my knowledge and involvement in CPI grew, so did my career in Navy Medicine. While stationed at the Navy Bureau of Medicine and Surgery (BUMED) as a captain, I saw the impact of process improvement on headquarters-level policy development and execution firsthand. It is one thing for a hospital CEO or a Navy senior executive to say that he or she wants CPI to be implemented; it is far different to create the push, the drive, or the motivation for it when the hospital staff is overwhelmed with the everyday work of taking care of patients. That drive or powerful motivation must come from on high. If the executive leadership doesn't create the buy-in and make it important, no one else will either.

BUMED understood its role and responsibility in the top-down leadership for Navy Medicine. This later served me well as I progressed to executive officer and then commanding officer in Navy Medicine. It became my responsibility to *walk the talk* and use my own top-down approach to accelerate CPI throughout my commands. I was keenly aware that the moment I stopped leading the effort—the moment I downplayed its importance—every physician, registered nurse, technician, and administrator on my staff would know that my words had been hollow. Fortunately, I was true to my words, and the staff expanded their CPI efforts to as many areas as possible. The results were impressive: Processing of administrative work was reduced by 50 percent, turnaround times for implementing specialty work was reduced by at least 45 percent, and orientation of new staff was accelerated by at least 35 percent, thus enabling them to begin their work far sooner than previously. I learned firsthand never to underestimate the power of senior leadership in leading anything that is important. The staff wants to do what is right, especially as it affects their work and their patients. Staff members need to know that their leader cares and will take the time, effort, and commitment to actually be a leader. My experience of 44 years in healthcare has been that in the eyes of employees, anything *less* is unacceptable!

As I transitioned to private-sector healthcare executive leadership, everything that I learned while in government became even more pronounced. Everyone is short on time: physicians, nursing staff, technicians, and administrators alike. Everyone is overloaded with work responsibilities. It was my job as a senior executive, working with other members of the executive suite, to not waste people's time. Serving as a champion for a performance-improvement team takes concentrated time, effort, and discipline. I knew that teams would not have unlimited time to use the tools to solve the tough problems they had been handed. It became my job to maximize whatever time was available—to focus the team's efforts as diligently as possible. What I learned from the private sector is that instilling teamwork, developing a common goal, and using the right people from the start are my job. As a senior executive, I could not delegate that work. Nor did I want to. The team's success was my success, and vice versa.

NOVACES has taken me farther than I ever dreamed. My recent work has enabled me to expand my skills and knowledge to fully understand the rigor and discipline of performance improvement, especially in the areas of Lean, Six Sigma, and Constraints Management. Improving healthcare's processes incrementally may be fine for solving the easy problems. Tackling the difficult ones, however, requires the diligent use of all three of these methodologies in a highly refined manner that leads to long-term sustainment.

One of several great lessons I have learned from my early days in TQM is that *sustainment* must be pursued vigorously. In other words, never let up! Another equally important lesson is about the use of data. Physicians, nurses, administrators, technicians, and executive leaders all use data to make decisions in their daily work. Along with my fellow colleagues, I, too, must continually use data to solve the tough, stubborn problems that we all face in today's healthcare environment. To not treat data with the importance it is due reduces my chances of success. In summary, what I've witnessed is the tremendous impact we can have by using the tools and methods of process improvement on our hospitals, patients and their families, our staff, and the entire healthcare community.

Captain Charles Mount shares his invaluable point of view based on his unique experience in military and civilian healthcare. Having spent almost four decades in military healthcare, Charles served at all four of Navy Medicine's large regional medical centers as the commanding officer of the Navy's Medical Sciences Training Command before he went on to become a for-profit hospital's chief nursing officer. His unrelenting optimism and positive energy combines with his leadership savvy to tackle the problems plaguing healthcare systems effectively.

In the course of writing this book, each of us has been a patient more than once. We have observed the vast numbers of inefficiencies, bottlenecks, and mistakes and the huge amounts of waste as both patients and practitioners. Every doctor, nurse, technician, administrator, and staff member is a patient at some point. Every year when health insurance renewal time comes, we all continue to be frustrated with rising costs and diminishing benefits, from individual consumers to small business owners and large corporations. There are few issues that touch so many lives as the importance of quality healthcare.

We are all on the same boat. The state of healthcare today is not unlike the engine room of that cargo ship I was aboard over 30 years ago, where everything was breaking down. Putting out the fire is no longer enough, for each spark alights a new blaze. It does not have to be this way. Proven tools and methods are now available to attack root causes of systemic problems rather than putting Band-Aids on symptoms. These techniques empower teams to develop practical solutions to achieve better quality of care while containing costs. And just as critical as achieving those improvements is the sustainment of those gains, lest all the effort expended in the name of performance improvement be for naught. What it will take to make this happen is described in this book. There is a better solution on the horizon— and in the pages ahead.

Bahadir Inozu, Ph.D.
Chief Executive Officer and Cofounder
NOVACES, LLC

ACKNOWLEDGMENTS

We could not have produced this book without the contributions of our colleagues at NOVACES, LLC. We would like to thank first and foremost, our research associate, Jeremy Schwartz, for his passion, assistance, and tireless dedication. We also would like to thank to Ivan Radovic and Brian MacClaren, cofounders of NOVACES, for their support.

In addition, we would like to thank Chris Zephro, Dr. Kevin Watson, Jan Bauer, Chuck Gaster, Suzanne Roberts, and the rest of the NOVACES family, as well as Tommy Houston, Brian McCormack, and Zina Amin, for their contributions.

We also thank our clients as well as Dr. Will Millhiser, Dr. Kelvyn Youngman, Dr. Emre Veral, Dr. Seza Gulec, Dr. Gary S. Wadhwa, Dr. Burak Acar, Dr. Hasan Kuş, Dr. Metin Çakmakçı, Henry Camp of IDEA, LLC, Michael Pitcher of Operations Excellence Consulting, Inc., John Wiley & Sons, Inc., The Commonwealth Fund, Theory of Constraints Certification Organization, and the late Dr. Eliyahu Goldratt whose teachings changed countless lives and are helping to create a more harmonious and prosperous world. Special thanks are due to Dr. Robert Halder and Dr. Hulusi Cinar for reviewing this book. Finally, we would like to thank to our families, friends, and colleagues who so faithfully supported the intent of this book and our efforts. We are in your debt.

Bahadir Inozu
Dan Chauncey
Vickie Kamataris
Charles Mount

Performance
Improvement
for Healthcare

CHAPTER 1

Performance Improvement in Healthcare

These Are the Best of Times, These Are the Worst of Times . . .

No not *that* book! We are talking about the state of healthcare not just in the United States but around the world. Even though we are at the forefront of the most advanced ability to heal, a great many people are deprived of the best of care either because they cannot afford it or because they are otherwise denied access to treatment. This book is not about the social aspects of that state but about what every healthcare leader and his or her organization can do to make healthcare more available, more affordable, with better outcomes . . . and yes, if desired, more profitable.

The United States spends more on healthcare than any other nation in the world, yet 50.7 million people in the United States have no health coverage. In 2008, $7,681 was spent for every U.S. resident on healthcare, some $2.3 trillion, as reported by the Centers for Medicare and Medicaid Services, yet the average life expectancy in the United States is shorter than that in many developed and developing nations. In a study of the healthcare systems of seven industrialized countries, the Commonwealth Fund ranked the U.S. healthcare system as the most costly, spending almost twice as much per capita than average.

How can this be?

The healthcare system in the United States is in shambles. Emergency departments are overflowing with the uninsured. There is a shortage of primary care providers driven by lifestyle and reimbursement pressures and a rush to specialize. The Affordable Care Act could extend health insurance coverage to 32 million uninsured U.S. citizens. There are fears that there won't be enough doctors to treat the newly insured because the United States could face a deficit of as many as 150,000 doctors in the next 15 years, according to the Association of American Medical Colleges. Like doctors, nurses have been working more overtime and take care of more and more patients, leading to the exit of experienced nurses from the profession because of burnout and exhaustion. Forty percent of practicing nurses are 50 years old or older. In the journal *Health Affairs*, Rother and Lavizzo-Mourey project that within the next 15 years, the U.S. nursing shortage will reach a shortfall of 260,000 registered nurses. Dedicated physicians and nurses are already working against impossible odds to achieve improbable results. How will care be provided to this expanding population of patients?

The answer is *not* by working harder.

The United States has more modern hospitals, more skilled physicians, more specialists, and more professional nurses than any other nation in the world. Most of the advances in healthcare technology, pharmacology, and medical science have originated in the United States. Applicants to medical schools in the United States compete with applicants from other nations seeking the world's best medical education. The American Recovery and Reinvestment Act (ARRA) of 2009 allocated about $30 billion to develop a national health information technology (IT) infrastructure. Yet the expected return on investment in technology, unlike advances in pharmacology and medical science, has not been fully realized. In the book *Curing Health Care: New Strategies for Quality Improvement*, Dr. Donald Berwick and colleagues wrote, "[T]ens of billions of dollars have gone into IT systems in healthcare, . . . but patients and care providers have very little to show for it."

The answer is *not* by spending more.

What Is the Answer?

If working harder and spending more is not the answer, what is? Healthcare systems are full of waste and experience an enormous amount of variation and many preventable mistakes. Furthermore, constraints and bottlenecks need careful management to get the most value for the money spent. The ailments of healthcare today are comorbid. Hence a direct, concentrated triage of the system is needed.

Other afflicted industries have found effective remedies for similar challenges. While acknowledging the uniqueness of humans and the complexity of healthcare delivery, three industrially based methodologies have been applied successfully in healthcare systems worldwide to achieve dramatic results. These are

1. **Lean**—a systematic approach to eliminate waste
2. **Six Sigma**—a rigorous, data-driven process to reduce variation and eradicate defects
3. **Constraints Management**—a breakthrough methodology to focus efforts and manage a system's bottlenecks and other constraints

Of the three, Lean applications in healthcare appear to be the most popular among U.S. and U.K. hospitals. More than 50 percent of hospitals in the United Kingdom are reporting the implementation of Lean methodology related to service improvement in their 2007 and 2008 annual reports. Six Sigma applications follow closely. According to an American Society for Quality (ASQ) survey of 77 hospitals, of about 5,000 hospitals nationwide, 53 percent apply Lean and 42 percent apply Six Sigma at some level, and 37 percent take the hybrid approach of Lean Six Sigma. On the other hand, Constraints Management applications in healthcare are at their infancy in the United States, but breakthroughs by effectively managing constraints are documented at hospitals in the United Kingdom, Israel, the Netherlands, South Africa, Singapore, and New Zealand.

Although each of these methodologies has its merits, a careful integration of them promises much more effective results than practicing any single methodology in isolation. For healthcare executives and midlevel managers who are dissatisfied with the status quo of hospital operations in terms of patient outcomes and experience, financial viability, and employee satisfaction, this book offers a best of breed integration of the latest advances in performance-improvement approaches.

A healthcare system is complex and composed of many subsystems with many interdependent processes. It includes payers, providers, inpatients, outpatients, and ancillary services, to name a few. A systems thinker sees a hospital "not as the sum of its parts, but primarily as the product of its interactions," as Dr. Russell Ackoff originally wrote and as the book *The Nun and the Bureaucrat* described. While the goal is to boost performance across healthcare organizations, the path is through identifying system constraints and improving the processes associated with them that are not meeting expectations. Unlike *one size fits all* or dogmatic approaches, such as Lean *only* or Six Sigma *only* or Constraints Management *only*, an integrated approach uses these three methodologies and others. By focusing on what is critical to the organization and by using the right tool for the right problem at the right time, faster results and greater return on investment can be realized—especially in these turbulent times.

The pace of change in healthcare is accelerating. Better tools are needed to provide front-line staff with the ability to better respond to those changes. Adaptation is happening, but just not fast enough to keep pace with the times. Currently, hospitals tend to use find-organize-clarify-understand-select (FOCUS)–plan-do-check-act (PDCA) supplemented, in some instances, with an industrial engineering approach to performance improvement. This outside-in approach allows only a minimal involvement of clinical staff. These are the individuals who do the work, know the process, deal with the problems, and need to be a part of the solution.

The problems with and the solutions to the healthcare crisis are not about people nor technology nor science. They are about transforming the system. Fifty percent of $2.3 trillion spent per year on healthcare in the United States is wasted because of inefficient processes. Therefore, the answer is to fix the *system* of inefficient processes, to prevent mistakes, and to manage the bottlenecks better by focusing on the right problem with the right tool at the right time—in other words, to use an integrated approach to performance improvement.

Is it possible for a hospital to improve outcomes while improving its performance as a business at the same time?

It's All About . . . the Patient . . . the Money— Why Not Both?

At the end of the day, when all is said and done, performance improvement is all about doing what is right for one patient while ensuring that the organization has the resources to continue doing what is right for the next patient. The entire healthcare industry is in the business of providing the right care to the right patients at the right time and in the right place. Performance improvement is about making that possible. As one hospital CEO put it: "Hospitals are a business; they are in the business of caring for patients and families. I'm here to help my hospital's business of improving the quality of care to my patients wherever and whenever possible." In *Managing in the Next Society*, management professor, writer, and guru Peter Drucker declared that "health care is the most difficult, chaotic, and complex industry to manage today" and that the hospital is "altogether the most complex human organization ever devised."

Healthcare professionals have been trained to provide care, and many of them have internalized it as their chosen vocation—not just *a job*. It is what gets them excited—ready to get up each day to devote their time, energy, and expertise. Physicians, nurses, technicians, healthcare administrators—all have prepared themselves during their early college and postgraduate years for learning how a hospital functions, how to render high-quality medical and nursing care to the sick, and how to maximize the most effective use of their skills. Now they are being told that they must factor in costs in a significant way. It is often difficult for healthcare professionals to internalize the business aspects of patient care.

Healthcare is an intensely competitive business climate. Given that, is improving the quality of patient care compatible with reducing costs? Is it possible on the one hand to increase the hospital's clinical outcomes or performance and still improve business performance? Examples of clinical outcomes or performance include

▲ Reducing patient falls
▲ Reducing pressure ulcers
▲ Reducing readmissions
▲ Decreasing hospital-acquired infections
▲ Decreasing inappropriate lengths of stay

The question becomes: Should attention be paid to these outcome improvements or to cost savings? Then again, maybe this question is moot.

The Cost and Quality in Healthcare

Recent changes in reimbursement for pressure ulcers make addressing this issue critical. Knapp Medical Center in Weslaco, Texas, attributes approximately $2.8 million in savings through performance improvement. In one year, Knapp's reductions in average length of stay resulted in eliminating 1,304 days of unnecessary care. The hospital also saved 98 days through eliminating readmissions, 27 deaths were prevented, and it avoided complications in 28 patients.

Hospital-acquired infections is another area that recent changes in reimbursement have affected. In an article from *Hospital Topics*, Hassan and colleagues estimated that a hospital-acquired infection increases the hospital care cost of a patient by $10,375, and it increases the length of stay by 3.30 days. These costs vary based on the nature of the infection, ranging from $600 for a urinary tract infection to $50,000 for prolonged bloodstream infection. Overall, medical errors add huge costs to the delivery of care. An examination of patient safety indicators (PSIs) showed that 90-day expenditures that are likely attributable to PSIs ranged from $646 for iatrogenic problems (i.e., accidental lacerations, pneumothorax, and so on) to $28,218 for acute respiratory failure, with up to 20 percent of these costs incurred after discharge. With a third of all 90-day deaths occurring after discharge, the excess death rate associated with PSIs ranged from 0 to 7 percent. The excess 90-day readmission rate associated with PSIs ranged from 0 to 8 percent. Overall, 11 percent of all deaths, 2 percent of readmissions, and 2 percent of expenditures likely were due to these PSIs. In a *Health Services Research* article, William Encinosa and Fred Hellinger posit that medical error studies that focus only on the inpatient stay can underestimate the impact of patient safety events by up to 20 to 30 percent.

Linking outcomes and patient safety to cost is at the forefront of current healthcare literature. What about the broader link between quality management and organizational performance—specifically, financial performance? In a recent study entitled, "Impact of Quality Management on Hospital Performance: An Empirical Examination," in *Quality Management Journal*, Carter and colleagues clearly demonstrated the connection. While the broader association between product or service quality and cost across virtually all industries is widely accepted and supported in the literature, the relationship as it pertains directly to healthcare was examined in an analysis of 175 hospitals. In addition to the link itself, the possible moderating effects of environmental uncertainty and hospital size were studied. The study found that there was a relationship between quality management and organization performance. While this is not surprising—and supports findings across most industries—there were a couple of additional conclusions worth addressing.

The first is that hospital size did make a difference in the strength of the relationship between quality management and organization performance. The relationship is not as strong for larger hospitals perhaps because of the need for smaller hospitals to pay attention to performance issues—both quality and financial. Despite their limited resources, smaller hospitals take a more strategic approach to quality as opposed to relying on more ad hoc practices.

The second conclusion is that environmental uncertainty also has a moderating effect. In examining the effects of environmental uncertainty, including factors such as government regulations, the financial market, the general economy, and public opinion, it was found that there was a stronger relationship between quality management and organization performance during times of low environmental uncertainty. The authors of the study posited that during times of high environmental uncertainty, leadership focus is diverted away from quality management to what the leaders view as more pressing issues.

Carter and colleagues summarize their findings by stating, ". . . it is important for managers in the healthcare community to include both quality practices and quality context in their quality management activities to improve overall hospital performance based on financial performance, market development, and quality outcomes."

On a final note about the financial issues facing healthcare in general and hospitals more specifically, *New York Magazine* published an article detailing the history and demise of St. Vincent's Hospital. St. Vincent's had accumulated $1 billion in debt and was losing $10 million per month. Having treated victims from the time of the *Titanic* through 9/11, nothing could save this landmark hospital. Neither could the fact that it was the only hospital on Manhattan's West Side below 59th Street and left 200,000 New Yorkers without their community hospital, as shown in Figure 1.1. As a result of financial mismanagement, St. Vincent's was closed on April 30, 2010. It was the seventeenth hospital to close in New York City since 2000. From an outcomes perspective, there is one certainty: Hospitals cannot provide quality care if they are closed!

The History of Performance Improvement in Healthcare

"Those who cannot remember the past are condemned to repeat it."

—GEORGE SANTAYANA, SPANISH-AMERICAN
PHILOSOPHER AND WRITER

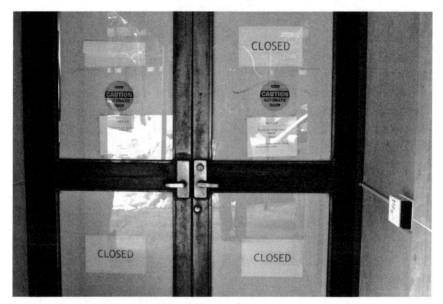

Figure 1.1 Closed doors of St. Vincent's Hospital.

Florence Nightingale

In order to better understand where we are today, it is helpful to revisit the evolution of performance improvement in healthcare. Its genesis can be traced back to the efforts of Florence Nightingale and her team. As Neuhauser recounted in *Florence Nightingale: A Passionate Statistician*, in November of 1854, Nightingale and her team of 38 nurses arrived at the British hospital in Üsküdar on the Asian side of Istanbul, Turkey, to care for the soldiers wounded in the Crimean War (1853–1856). When they arrived, they found the sanitary conditions of the hospital to be totally unsatisfactory. A British soldier had a better chance of surviving the war than surviving the filthy conditions of the hospital. Infectious diseases killed more soldiers than war wounds. A passionate statistician, Nightingale recorded that in the first seven months of the campaign, 60 percent of the soldiers died from infections. She and her team focused on improving cleanliness, sanitation, nutrition, administrative order, and patient care.

In the following three years, Nightingale and her team drastically improved the conditions for the care of soldiers, reducing the death rate among patients by two-thirds. Her careful data collection, analysis and reasoned conclusions were instrumental in her success, along with her leadership skills. With aristocratic connections and established access to funding and media, Nightingale enjoyed the support of top leadership, Queen Victoria. Her book, *Notes on Hospitals*, is credited as the only book on modern hospital management in the nineteenth century. Her recommendations influenced hospitals worldwide. Building on Nightingale's achievements, many others contributed to the evolution of performance improvement in healthcare, such as Ernest Codman, W. Edwards Deming, Walter Shewhart, Avedis Donabedian, and Joseph Juran.

In the fall of 1987, Dr. Donald Berwick and the aforementioned Juran launched the National Demonstration Project (NDP) as a new and rigorous approach to improving hospital performance with Total Quality Management (TQM), a variant of Continuous Quality Improvement (CQI). Twenty-one American healthcare organizations joined as members of the NDP. Hosted by the Harvard Community Health Plan, project participants experimented with using TQM tools, which were being implemented successfully by other industry leaders such as Toyota, Mitsubishi, Honda, Sony, Xerox, and Motorola. Their findings were summarized in *Curing Health Care: New Strategies for Quality Improvement*. Some of the NDP hospitals succeeded with respectable results. As the success stories of NDP spread, numerous other hospital CEOs started experimenting with TQM. However, although Berwick was quoted as saying that as many as 1,000 U.S. hospitals had begun TQM efforts, he did qualify by saying, "But I'd be surprised if there are 100 that are really serious." Dr. Berwick later transformed the NDP into the Institute for Healthcare Improvement (IHI).

Naval Medicine

The Naval Regional Medical Center San Diego (NRMC SD), which is the U.S. Navy's largest hospital, and the Navy Bureau of Medicine & Surgery (BUMED) were key members of the NDP from 1989 to 1995. In 1989, Vice Admiral James Zimble, the Navy Surgeon General at BUMED, introduced TQM to his commanding officers. Rear Admiral Robert Halder, the commanding officer of NMSC SD, was a participant at this introductory meeting. Rear Admiral Halder indicated that he was ready to lead a very ambitious deployment of TQM for his command of 5,000 employees and eight other region-wide hospitals. He wrote, "This was what I had been looking for. . . . I was leading a good organization—but this was the way to make it great." Both Zimble and Halder saw the promise of TQM and CQI, understood the FOCUS-PDCA model, and knew that healthcare, in general, had to change all across the spectrum. They stepped out quickly, and Navy Medicine became a vigorous proponent of TQM throughout the NDP.

The military embraced Total Quality Management (TQM) in 1988 throughout the Army, Navy, Air Force, and Marine Corps. In 1990, the Chief of Naval Operations changed the Navy's use of TQM to Total Quality Leadership (TQL) to emphasize the critical importance of leadership in improving any process. TQM or TQL was considered an overarching cornerstone and became almost synonymous with Continuous Quality Improvement (CQI).

To ensure that it would not become a fleeting flavor-of-the-month program, in 1989, Rear Admiral Halder set up a separate office at the NRMC SD to focus completely on the transformation to TQL. To demonstrate highest-level leadership of this transformation, Rear Admiral Halder required the TQL office director, then-Commander Charles Mount, one of this book's coauthors, to report directly to him, thereby bypassing the normal bureaucratic layers in Navy Medicine. These two officers met each morning at 7 A.M. TQL success was the top priority. The goal was to have the TQL office operate in coordination with the NRMC SD's traditional Quality Assurance and Improvement (QA&I) Department. Interestingly, both areas were directed to work hand in hand to bring the concepts of CQI to all levels of hospital staff, especially those who actually touched the patients (in Navy terms, this was called the *deck plate*). This was a novel approach. In previous years, the quality assurance functions were performed by a few QA&I experts at the directorate or department level. It was only during times of inspection by the Joint Commission on Accreditation of Healthcare Organizations that QA&I activities reached down to the department level. Since the TQL and QA&I offices complemented each other, the concepts of performance improvement became widespread among the hospital staff.

Implementing CQI at such a large medical center required more than just creating a TQL office. Training was provided to hundreds, if not thousands, of healthcare professionals. No one hospital could create such a large training system. To create such a system would require participation by numerous San Diego area hospitals. Rear Admiral Halder also asked Commander Charles Mount to gain that participation by creating a community-wide coalition. The

Naval Regional Medical Center offered direction and support, inviting the CEOs of 26 hospitals in the San Diego area and the commanding officers of the 6 Navy hospitals to form the Southern California Coalition for Improving Health Care Quality. Rear Admiral Halder told them, "I cannot do this alone. I need you to join me."

Twenty-four civilian and military hospitals chose to join the Southern California Coalition for Improving Healthcare when it commenced in November 1989. During the first three years of deployment at NRMC SD, the cumulative success of over 60 teams working on both administrative and clinical processes yielded a cost reduction of $22 million while significantly improving internal and external customer satisfaction and quality of care at the same time. Similar successes were achieved by many of the coalition's civilian facilities. Ultimately, thousands of patients were positively affected by the work of the coalition. The coalition lasted until 1995, sponsoring numerous CQI conferences in San Diego and fulfilling its mission of acculturating hospitals with the tools, methodologies, and training to sustain CQI. Attendees at the conferences included healthcare professionals from across the United States.

What's in a Name?

While the name fluctuated between TQM, TQL, CQI, and Continuous Process Improvement (CPI) and a relative amount of success was achieved, hospital executives in the United States were becoming dissatisfied, according to a survey conducted in 1992. Initially in separate offices, as staffing issues arose, most hospitals integrated TQM and CQI into the hospitals' QA&I offices. The goal was to conserve resources and place all process-improvement activities in a single area under a single leader or manager. Unfortunately, many QA&I offices were already overloaded with Joint Commission initiatives, reporting quality indicators, Healthcare Effectiveness Data and Information Set (HEDIS) measures, risk management and safety functions, and attending and taking minutes at myriad committee meetings. Larger hospitals could afford to hire sufficient personnel to divide up such tasks. Smaller hospitals reduced the QA&I staffing to one to three people. Thus the attention needed to sustain these TQM or CQI efforts was diverted elsewhere, diminishing overall effectiveness.

As has been the Joint Commission's philosophy for more than 20 years, it promoted the CPI or performance-improvement moniker. In so doing, it wanted to foster the collaborative use of toolsets, whatever they are titled, throughout the entire hospital structure and ultimately to see results that improve patient outcomes. Specifically, the Joint Commission was interested in nursing, medical, and ancillary personnel working together as a team rather than in silos, as they had functioned traditionally. Only by working in a cooperative atmosphere, the Joint Commission surmised, would hospitals gain any traction in solving persistent problems and actually improve patient-care processes. At the tactical level, Deming's plan-do-check-act (PDCA) cycle had arisen as the primary improvement approach. As described in the following section, PDCA (also referred to as plan-do-study-act, or PDSA) is no longer sufficient to address the performance-improvement challenges of today's hospitals as healthcare costs skyrocket.

FOCUS-PDCA

"The definition of insanity is doing the same thing over and over again and expecting different results."

—ALBERT EINSTEIN

Although plan-do-check-act (PDCA) was developed originally by the father of statistical quality control, Walter A. Shewhart, W. Edwards Deming, who was his student, later went on to develop Total Quality Management (TQM) and became a founding father of management science in his own right. Deming's application of PDCA (and PDSA) called for managers to hypothesize, develop, and *plan* improvements; implement and *do* the improvements, almost as if performing a scientific experiment; *checking*, studying, and evaluating the outcomes and results; and then *acting* based on considered analysis to instill the change on a continued basis until it could be improved further. In so doing, Deming applied the principles of scientific management to the aim of perpetually improving organizations. Supplementing PDCA with FOCUS, Hospital Corporation of America added yet another acronym to the vernacular—find-organize-clarify-understand-select (FOCUS). In the FOCUS-PDCA paradigm, preceding PDCA, FOCUS calls for *finding* an improvement opportunity, *organizing* an improvement team, *clarifying* the current state of the process, *understanding* the causes for variation in the process, and *selecting* the improvement.

Is the traditional FOCUS-PDCA sufficient to truly solve today's healthcare problems and transform the industry? Hospitals have long used the tools and methodologies of FOCUS-PDCA for performance improvement. Hospital Corporation of America (HCA) adapted Deming's PDCA and added the FOCUS portion specifically to help hospitals select their most inefficient and troublesome areas for improvement. This methodology was started in the late 1980s and has been expanded across the entire industry over the past 20 years.

If PDCA were sufficient, then the United States would not be in a healthcare crisis. The United States has the most costly healthcare system in the world, and its performance ranks poorly in comparison with other countries. In a study where the United States and six other industrialized countries (Australia, Canada, Germany, the Netherlands, New Zealand, and the United Kingdom) were compared, the United States ranked last or next-to-last in all five of the primary dimensions considered:

▲ Quality care
▲ Access
▲ Efficiency
▲ Equity
▲ Long, healthy, productive lives

These poor rankings by the United States have been consistent in the 2004, 2006, 2007, and 2010 studies. The United States pays dearly for its poor performance, with per capita expenditures far exceeding those in the other countries, as shown in Figure 1.2. These monetary costs do not take

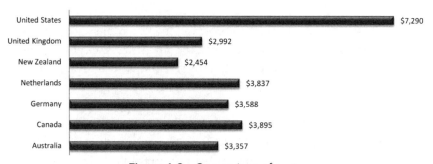

Figure 1.2 Comparison of costs.

into account the unquantifiable value of human life and patient satisfaction squandered by an underperforming healthcare system.

FOCUS-PDCA continues to be used by many hospitals as the primary performance-improvement approach they employ to meet the requirements of the Joint Commission for its three-year accreditations. The Joint Commission's mission is to improve the safety and quality of care provided to the public through the provision of healthcare accreditation and related services that support performance improvement in healthcare organizations. While the Joint Commission does not mandate which methodology is used, it has included Lean and Six Sigma as methodologies to improve its own internal processes. Joint Commission President Dr. Mark Chassin is a certified Lean Six Sigma practitioner.

Historically, FOCUS-PDCA has shown some degree of success in improving healthcare processes. Still, most of these successes have been reactive in nature and generally have not improved financial results. FOCUS-PDCA does not cultivate the breakthroughs for which an integrated approach to performance improvement is ideally suited. In essence, it is no longer adequate. For example, at Seattle Children's Hospital, staff would stockpile supplies. A nurse in the intensive-care unit (ICU) was concerned about having the tools she needed for her patients, so she began stashing them away. The hoarding of supplies in the ICU was the tipping point in creating supply-chain issues, which correspondingly resulted in even more shortages. This is the type of problem that is not normally addressed by FOCUS-PDCA. FOCUS-PDCA does not yield the breakthroughs that are being realized by an integrated approach to performance improvement.

No Quick Fix   Today's healthcare processes involve extensively broken or misplaced steps with multiple handoffs, too many decision points, and a host of inadequately managed constraints. If they can be resolved with traditional FOCUS-PDCA, then all is well and good. Typically, however, all is not well. For so many of today's hospitals, the improvements are often short-lived and require endless rework. Deming saw this situation repeated over and over again across many industries. He cautioned against reaching for the quick fix or Band-Aid but rather encouraged a walk through the entire process. The primary fault lies not with the hospital staff. Quite frankly, no individual or group of people is at fault. No matter how hard people try, until the underlying system is fixed, sustained improvement will be impossible.

In their article, "Moving Quality to the Top of the Hospital Agenda," Byrnes and Fifer state that a quiet revolution is taking place that places quality improvement and overall performance improvement as the link between better outcomes (i.e., patient safety and delivery of care) and lower costs. This revolution includes the allocation of resources for quality programs and the discussion of quality at the operational meetings of executive leadership teams.

Despite this increased level of activity in performance improvement, improvements are not being sustained. There are at least three reasons for this:

▲ Time pressures create the desire for fast solutions.
▲ Attention spans are short and easily overcome by tomorrow's priorities.
▲ Problems cut across multiple departments with no single owner of the process.

What is needed, then, is a methodology that is sufficient to achieve true sustainment. It must be robust, involve disciplined thinking, and focus heavily on data. It therefore must be strong enough to break through healthcare's *hidden factory* and uncover the true cost of poor quality. This is illustrated in Figure 1.3.

What lies above the waterline in Figure 1.3 is where much of the day-to-day performance improvements are focused:

▲ Inventory difficulties
▲ Treatment errors
▲ Redundant tests
▲ Lost revenue

What lies *below* the waterline are all the issues that prevent processes from being resolved permanently, including such items as long cycle times, unused capacity, planning delays, and excessive employee turnover. Because they are below the water surface and thus hidden, they exhibit five characteristics that are difficult to resolve:

▲ Murky and therefore challenging to readily see
▲ Deep and complex, requiring advanced tools
▲ Tough to extract, entrenched as if stuck in the muck of a river bed

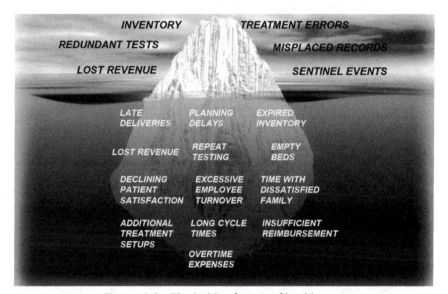

INVENTORY   TREATMENT ERRORS

REDUNDANT TESTS   MISPLACED RECORDS

LOST REVENUE   SENTINEL EVENTS

LATE   PLANNING   EXPIRED
DELIVERIES   DELAYS   INVENTORY

LOST REVENUE   REPEAT   EMPTY
          TESTING   BEDS

DECLINING   EXCESSIVE   TIME WITH
PATIENT   EMPLOYEE   DISSATISFIED
SATISFACTION   TURNOVER   FAMILY

ADDITIONAL   LONG CYCLE   INSUFFICIENT
TREATMENT   TIMES   REIMBURSEMENT
SETUPS
          OVERTIME
          EXPENSES

Figure 1.3 The hidden factory of healthcare.

▲ Rarely, if ever, come to the surface for easy analysis
▲ Loaded with multiple other problems and difficult to break apart into bite-sized chunks

FOCUS-PDCA has not shown that it is capable of breaking through the hidden factory. A reactive approach only works sporadically and results in limited long-term sustainability, which is far less than optimal. An integrated performance-improvement deployment has sufficient rigor to assess the issues below the water line accurately and raise the dangerous and most inefficient or costly processes to the surface, where they can be resolved. Without a structured and rigorous performance-improvement program that is supported by the executive leadership team, many broken healthcare processes remain that way. Occasionally, they rise to the surface for a fast fix, only to sink back down into the submergence of the hidden factory.

For example, trying to improve patient flow in the Emergency Department (ED) can be a daunting undertaking. There are multiple departments; a host of physicians, nurses, technicians, and clerks involved; and exhaustive resources required to manage multiple flows. In such a complex system, quality and cost issues are sure to be present. When they do arise, time constraints tend to result in temporary fixes instead of more enduring solutions that make fundamental changes in root causes. Initially, the issue appears to be resolved: The flow of patients improves or the quality issue seems to be fixed. However, it is only a matter of time before the quick fix unravels, and the patient flow reverts back to its original state or the same quality issue resurfaces.

True sustainment requires a permanent fix—a fundamental change to the underlying process. That is the weakness of FOCUS-PDCA as it has evolved in healthcare today. While the basic theory does provide for the requisite rigor, it lacks a documented application process, as well as specific application of the tools necessary to drive both quality and financial improvements at both the process and system levels. Rather than being a failure of the intent behind PDCA, its failure lies in a lack of a *rigorous* process mandating the commitment of upper management to enforce the suggested procedures. Soft skills were not given the attention that they deserved to manage change successfully. There are so many stakeholders prevalent in healthcare processes, and prior improvement methods did not have the capability to achieve the buy-in necessary to initialize and sustain the change. Instead of being taken as a responsibility of management itself, performance improvement was relegated to a separate silo: the Quality Department.

The move to improve the quality and cost-effectiveness of healthcare is gaining momentum due to its skyrocketing costs. Healthcare reform is being debated widely regarding its efficacy in its current form. In his *ASQ Quality Progress* article, Edmund states that quality and patient safety advocates say that it will help to improve quality of care, delivery of care, and patient safety. For healthcare organizations to keep their doors open, leadership must realize that both quality and financial performance must improve.

Complementary (Core) Methodologies

As TQM was losing its popularity in the manufacturing industry, Lean, Six Sigma, and Constraints Management, which is based on the theory of constraints (TOC), emerged as three schools of thought for performance improvement during the mid-1980s. By relegating these proven methodologies to only being applicable in manufacturing, healthcare delayed embracing them and thus adopted them even more slowly than other service and transactional industries.

Performance improvement in healthcare started to catch up with the other industries beginning in the early 1990s. The first application of Constraints Management in healthcare on record was at the University of Pretoria Medical School in 1991 in South Africa. Mount Carmel Health in Columbus, Ohio, was one of the first healthcare organizations to implement Six Sigma throughout its entire organization. Its Six Sigma deployment started in July 2000. Vickie Kamataris, one of this book's coauthors, applied Six Sigma in healthcare within General Electric for the first time in 1997. Her story appears in the Preface. In 2002, executives from Virginia Mason Medical Center visited Japan and began their journey to implementing Lean principles. Their success is encouraging other hospitals to implement Lean, especially in the United States and the United Kingdom.

Until the late 1990s, Lean, Six Sigma, and Constraints Management methodologies were like three different religions—coexisting but independent of each other. As late business process management pioneer and father of the swim-lane diagram, Dr. Geary Rummler, said, there are "turf wars between competing process-improvement philosophies, methodologies and technologies." Then Lean and Six Sigma were integrated and became the leading approach in the early 2000s, whereas integration of Lean and Constraints Management also were applied in manufacturing and defense. Constraints Management is arguably the least known among these three methodologies, especially in the U.S. healthcare industry. An informal survey conducted by NOVACES shows that very few U.S. hospital executives have even heard of Constraints Management.

On the other hand, Constraints Management applications have been resulting in major improvements in the hospitals of the United Kingdom, New Zealand, South Africa, Singapore, and Israel and is remarkably popular in Dutch healthcare. If a hospital in the Netherlands has a process-improvement methodology applied, then one-third chooses Constraints Management. Constraints Management is significantly more popular in Dutch hospitals than in Dutch manufacturing. Breakthrough potential is even greater when Constraints Management is carefully integrated with Lean and Six Sigma.

Three Windows: Constraints Management, Lean, and Six Sigma

Three methodologies—Six Sigma, Lean, and Constraints Management—have risen to the forefront and bridged the gap between manufacturing and service/transactional industries—especially the ever-expanding healthcare environment. These three approaches are very complementary. Lean and Six Sigma are primarily process-improvement approaches. On the other hand, Constraints Management takes a system perspective at a higher level by looking at the interdependencies among processes and their dynamics for system improvement.

When separated, Lean tools cannot bring a process under statistical control, and Six Sigma cannot improve cycle time dramatically, as Michael George states in his book, *Lean Six Sigma*. Lean promotes elimination of waste everywhere without necessarily a focus on the overall system, and Six Sigma has an inherent risk of local optimization. Constraints Management highlights where to *focus* improvement efforts for system-level impact by offering a dynamic holistic view where bottlenecks and the weakest links of healthcare organizations become not only visible but also manageable for maximum value. Lean and Six Sigma tools allow teams to produce solutions to better manage constraints. Constraints Management is excellent in providing a step-by-step approach to direct improvement efforts, but it does not tell you how to get the most mileage out of the bottleneck. Once the direction is set, Lean and Six Sigma tools help an organization reach its destination.

The integrated approach is analogous to looking through three windows into a system: Lean, Six Sigma, and Constraints Management windows. The Constraints Management window is like looking at the forest from a hot air balloon and selecting the best tree from which to pick fruit. The Lean window shows the simplest way to pick the low-hanging fruits as well as the fruit on the floor with very little effort. And the Six Sigma window shows how to consistently pick the bulk of the sweeter fruits, without bruising them, at higher, difficult-to-reach branches of the tree.

Essential principles of these three methodologies are introduced in this chapter. Since Constraints Management applications in healthcare are in their infancy, a more detailed description is provided in Chapter 2.

A Primer on Six Sigma and Its Applications in Healthcare

Traditionally, improvement of processes through a structured methodology largely has been the domain of industrial or quality engineers. Over the past two decades, a transition has taken place. Numerous methodologies have been implemented to operationalize performance improvement. Business Process Reengineering focused a great deal of emphasis on the use of technology in making processes more efficient. One set of philosophies focused on empowerment and worker involvement. Another focused on the importance of the use of tools and methods in conjunction with understanding the process.

W. Edwards Deming, along with others, began emphasizing the need to understand variation through the use of statistical tools such as Pareto and control charts. This latter concept, known as *Total Quality Management* (TQM), also shifted responsibility for quality improvement to those directly involved in the process. It was not until Six Sigma came along that all these concepts were combined into a single methodology. While Deming focused on the cultural transformation of businesses, other management pioneers, such as Joseph Juran and Philip Crosby, addressed the management and cost of quality, respectively. From Crosby's perspective, expenditures associated with improving quality should be offset by the resulting savings in warranties, scrap, rework, and other costs of poor quality.

Six Sigma has emerged as the primary vehicle for improving both manufacturing and service or transactional business processes. Six Sigma has been defined in many ways. The following definition, taken from *The Six Sigma Handbook,* by Thomas Pyzdek, is perhaps the most inclusive:

> Six Sigma is a rigorous and systematic methodology that utilizes information (management by facts) and statistical analysis to measure and improve a company's operational performance, practices and systems by identifying and preventing "defects" in manufacturing and service-related processes in order to anticipate and exceed expectations of all stakeholders to accomplish effectiveness.

Six Sigma applies a five-step method called Define-Measure-Analyze-Improve-Control (DMAIC). Each letter represents one of the steps in the methodology, as shown in Figure 1.4.

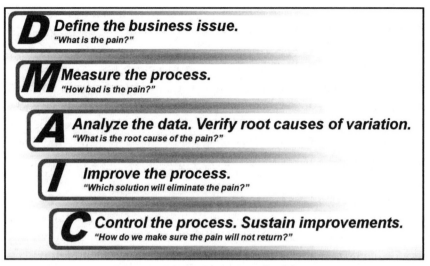

Figure 1.4 The DMAIC methodology.

The methodology includes the application of a full range of statistical tools yet recommends that it be implemented by teaching these statistical methods to workers throughout an organization—not limiting it to statisticians or industrial engineers. While the DMAIC methodology emphasizes the use of statistical tools, the strength is in the methodology itself. DMAIC is discussed further in Chapter 6.

Certain industries have been slower to accept certain quality tools and methods from manufacturing despite more than 50 years of successful application. It is critical to note that the finding is about acceptance, not applicability; for example, while control charts have been used extensively in manufacturing since the 1920s, they are slow to be accepted in direct patient care.

In healthcare, a Six Sigma project saves $500,000 annually, according to an article by David Frabatto in *Managed Healthcare*. However, in our experience, such claims cannot be taken for granted, but assuming that the project selection process is attuned, $500,000 or even more is achievable realistically. For example, a project within our deployment portfolio on a credentialing process for contracted healthcare workers resulted in validated savings of $789,000 per year and a replication potential to save an additional $114 million dollars. When a senior Six Sigma practitioner, called a Black

Belt, normally leads four to eight projects per year, annual savings from a single Six Sigma Black Belt could exceed $3 million dollars. As indicated by the positive financial impact that typically far surpasses its associated costs, quality improvement can be a major factor in a business's success.

It is very interesting that the same article in which Frabatto cited the $3 billion revenue gap also stated that New York hospitals would save $3.4 billion annually by reducing length of stay to national standards. Length of stay is just one performance gap where the root cause is unknown and where applying the right tool to the right problem at the right time makes a lot of sense.

The power of Six Sigma is its ability to identify root causes of complex problems and reduce variation, both of which are central to the improvement of processes. Examples of Six Sigma applications in healthcare include reduction of infection rates, patient falls, and missed appointments, as well as enhanced medication reconciliations and coding.

A Primer on Lean and Its Applications in Healthcare

Prior to the 1950s, one could argue that the United States *owned* the automobile market worldwide. Then, in 1950, a Japanese engineer named Eiji Toyoda spent three months at Ford's Rouge Plant in Detroit. This was the seminal point in the evolution of Lean. Between 1937 and 1950, Toyota had produced 2,685 automobiles total, compared with the almost 7,000 produced daily at the Rouge Plant.

In an effort to compete in the marketplace, Toyoda—along with others— adapted what he saw at Ford into the beginning of what came to be called the *Toyota Production System*. In 1990, Womack, Jones, and Roos coined the phrase *Lean Manufacturing*, and nothing has been the same ever since.

According to the Lean Enterprise Institute, Lean as a concept includes five basic principles:

- ▲ Specify value from the end customer's perspective.
- ▲ Identify all the steps in the value stream for each service, eliminating non-value-adding steps.
- ▲ Make the value-adding steps flow without interruption to the customer.
- ▲ Implement a pull system based on customer demand.
- ▲ As value is specified, value streams are identified, non-value-added steps are removed, and flow and pull are introduced, go back to back to step 1 and continue it until a state of perfection is reached with no waste.

In alignment with these principles, all processes should—*must*—add value to the customer, include only value-adding steps, and flow continuously from customer order to delivery. This *Lean archetype*, along with recognition that perfection is a journey, is equally applicable to manufacturing, services, and healthcare.

Efforts to apply Lean are focused on addressing specific issues or wastes. Seven *deadly wastes* have been identified. While these were developed originally for applicability within manufacturing, they are equally relevant in healthcare. An explanation of wastes as they relate to healthcare appears in Figure 1.5.

▲ **Transport.** Any time people, materials, or information must be moved, it is defined as waste. Moving patients from room to room is an example of waste. While in many cases necessary, this transportation nonetheless is viewed as waste. Use of a spaghetti diagram may help to minimize this type of waste.

▲ **Inventory.** While it is necessary to maintain inventories to ensure availability, anything short of just-in-time (JIT) availability is categorized as waste. Tools such as kanban can mitigate this kind of waste.

Wastes	Examples
Transport	1. Moving patients from room to room 2. Charts not centrally located 3. Poor layouts, lab located a long distance from the ED
Inventory	1. Overstocked medications on units/floors 2. Multiple locations for consumable goods 3. Multiple suppliers of surgical supplies 4. Any work in progress
Motion	1. Heavy items on top shelf, light items on bottom 2. Excessive bending, reaching, walking to complete a process step
Waiting	1. Specimens waiting analysis 2. Patients waiting to make appointments 3. Patients waiting to be seen for an appointment 4. Time lag with physician orders 5. Patients on hold for admission
Over-Production	1. Duplicate charting 2. Copies of reports sent automatically 3. Multiple forms with same information
Over-Processing	1. Clarifying orders 2. Increased size of patient records 3. Multiple blood specimen collections
Defects Requiring Rework or Scrap	1. Label on the wrong tube 2. Over/under coding 3. Decrease in revenue based on insurance claims 4. Decrease in patient satisfaction scores

Figure 1.5 The seven deadly wastes of Lean.

▲ **Motion.** A nurse's station with a desktop computer at one end and a printer at the other that requires nurses to move excessively to pick up printouts is an example of waste. Good ergonomic practices and more efficient workspace layouts can moderate this waste.

▲ **Waiting.** This waste is endemic to healthcare. We even call our primary customers patients—is this because it is an expectation? Elimination of non-value-adding activities can diminish this waste.

▲ **Overproduction.** Running too many tests and printing too many copies of paperwork are examples of overproduction. Reviewing standard lab panels or pursuing paperless processes can mitigate this type of waste.

▲ **Overprocessing.** Requiring excess approvals and running the same test twice are examples of overprocessing. The elimination of non-value-adding activities can lessen this sort of waste dramatically.

▲ **Defects.** When a product or service does not meet specification or customer expectations, it is a defect. Defects often result in rework, and the associated costs frequently go unaccounted for.

A *process-level value-stream analysis* (PVSA) and *rapid improvement workshop* (RIW) are often applied toward eliminating or reducing these wastes. These aspects will be addressed in much more detail in Chapter 6.

The power of Lean is its ability to eliminate waste and improve flow, which is central to the simplification of processes and reduction of delays and handoffs. Examples of Lean applications include reduction of non-value-added steps in the delivery of care, mistake-proofing hand sanitation, and standardizing referral management.

A Primer on Constraints Management

Constraints Management is a management philosophy encompassing an integrated suite of techniques used in operations and supply-chain management, project management, conflict resolution, and strategic planning. Dr. Eliyahu Goldratt began its development in 1979 with the production scheduling software OPT, and has led its evolution into three interrelated areas—logistics/production, performance measurement, and problem-solving/thinking tools.

The basic concepts of Constraints Management were introduced to the public as the theory of constraints in Goldratt's landmark book, *The Goal*. It was written as a novel, facilitating accessibility of the concepts to a wide audience. The text has been translated into over 21 languages, sold more than 5 million copies, and is still used to teach Constraints Management in college classrooms across the globe.

In *The Goal*, Goldratt details a systematic approach to managing complex organizations by identifying and controlling key leverage points within a system or process. By managing these key control points, healthcare organizations can focus on areas that drive system-level improvement instead of trying to manage every element of a process, which can lead to local optimization without systemic impact.

A *constraint* is anything that limits the system from achieving higher performance relative to its goal. In healthcare, a constraint is anything that impedes the ability or means to provide or deliver care. H. William Dettmer, author of numerous books on Constraints Management, defines seven basic constraint types:

▲ Market
▲ Resource
▲ Material
▲ Supplier/vendor
▲ Financial
▲ Knowledge/competence
▲ Policy

He also adds that a policy is most likely behind a constraint from any of the first six categories. On the other hand, Dr. Boaz Ronen, a business administration professor at Tel Aviv University and coauthor of the book, *Focused Operations Management for Health Services Organizations*, defines only four types of constraints in a managerial system:

▲ Resource
▲ Market
▲ Policy
▲ Dummy

The *Theory of Constraints International Certification Organization (TOCICO) Dictionary* calls policy constraint a common misnomer because "Bad policies are not the constraint; rather they hinder effective constraint management by inhibiting the ability to fully exploit and/or subordinate to the constraint." Regardless of how constraints are classified, the Constraints

Management body of knowledge provides tools to identify and manage all types of constraints.

Because of its simple yet robust methodology, Constraints Management has been applied to manufacturing, project management, retailing, supply-chain management, and process improvement with breakthrough results. A partial list of companies employing Constraints Management includes ABB, Delta Airlines, 3M, Amazon, Boeing, Ford Motor Company, Intel, and Microsoft; however, many Constraints Management adopters state an unwillingness to disclose improvements for competitive reasons. Not-for-profit and governmental organizations such as the British National Health Service, the United Nations, NASA, the U.S. Department of Defense, and the Israeli Air Force also have employed Constraints Management solutions successfully. Published studies from practitioners indicate that Constraints Management systems produce substantial benefits in terms of greater output while reducing inventory, manufacturing lead time, and the standard deviation of cycle time. Healthcare systems worldwide are learning a great deal about Constraints Management from these organizations.

Constraints Management is a *systems approach* that recognizes that every system has a goal and a set of necessary conditions that must be satisfied to achieve that goal. As such, Constraints Management begins by identifying the critical success factors necessary to realize the goal and aligns the system to attain greater levels of performance while minimizing waste. Goals may range from reaching superior levels of profitability now and in the future for a for-profit organization to increased coverage or availability of provided services for a not-for-profit company or government agency.

Because it is grounded in systems thinking, Constraints Management looks at materials, information, and money flows and encompasses techniques useful for production and logistics (e.g., drum-buffer-rope, critical chain project management, and buffer management), performance measurement (e.g., throughput accounting), and problem solving (e.g., thinking processes). It therefore breaks through the "silo mentality" of many organizations, focusing all efforts on satisfying end-user requirements. Dr. Kevin Watson of Iowa State University sees Constraints Management as focused, robust, scalable, and generalizable, as described in the next few paragraphs.

Constraints Management is *focused*, recognizing that the system's ability to attain its goal is inhibited by a limited set of variables or constraints.

Constraints Management focuses attention and concentrates resources at the point in the system where they may be leveraged to achieve the highest level of goal attainment. Constraints Management allows the system to achieve optimal output and increase flexibility and responsiveness, all while minimizing waste. This synergistic effect results from subordinating the system to the constraint and creating protective capacity at nonconstrained resources, thereby better enabling the system to deal with the consequences of variability.

Constraints Management tools are *robust*. Systems managed under Constraints Management strategically buffer against variability, do not impose rigid material-handling rules, and schedule only strategic control points in the system. Therefore, Constraints Management systems are better able to mitigate the effects of uncertainty than similar JIT systems. This makes Constraints Management adaptable for highly variable manufacturing and for the purpose of managing supply chains.

Constraints Management techniques are *scalable* and *generalizable* to a wide set of operations and supply-chain environments. Techniques that are useful at the process level are applicable at higher levels of aggregation. Constraints Management tools are also generalizable to applications far beyond production and logistics as they were presented originally in *The Goal*. The thinking processes used in the resolution of unstructured problems are applicable to decision making in such widely varying environments as conflict resolution, quality control, continuous improvement, contract negotiation, policy reengineering, and strategy development. Once managers understand the basic concepts, they are able to apply that knowledge with little additional training to a wide range of applications, for example, manufacturing and supply-chain environments—from control of a manufacturing cell, to project management, to distribution and logistics management.

Constraints Management Tools System improvements under Constraints Management seek to identify (1) what to change, (2) what to change to, and (3) how to cause the change. This follows a *process of ongoing improvement* (POOGI) comprised of two prerequisites and five steps that underlie all Constraints Management production techniques. The prerequisites for Constraints Management process improvement are (1) define the boundaries of the system and its goal, and (2) determine a means to measure goal attainment. While these steps appear obvious, failure to explicitly identify the scope and purpose of the system and measure how the system performs in achieving that goal can result in dysfunctional behavior. Having satisfied the prerequisites, system improvement proceeds according to the *five focusing steps* sequence:

1. *Identify* the system constraint(s). What limits the performance of the system now? What is the weakest link in the system?
2. Decide how to *exploit* the system's constraint(s). How can the most performance be achieved from a constrained step in the process without additional investment? Here, *exploit* means "use, develop, make use of, take advantage of, and make the most of."
3. *Subordinate/synchronize* everything else in the system to the above decision. Set up and implement rules to maximize the capacity of the system based on the speed of the system's constraint. In this step, all parts of the system that are *not* constraints are required to do whatever they can to support the exploitation plan. Additionally, all nonconstraints must not do anything that would interfere with the exploitation plan for the constraint. And most important, all nonconstraints (most of the system) must recognize that their own efficiency is not as important as supporting the system constraint, which requires measurement changes.
4. *Elevate* the system constraint. To physically increase the capacity of the system through the acquisition of or investment in more resources. Always remember to predict where the constraint will be after elevation and its resulting impact on global performance. The location of any new constraint definitely will affect an organization's elevate strategy.
5. *Go back* to step 1. This will ensure that improvement is ongoing and never ceases. It also helps to avoid inertia by keeping at bay the relentless tendency to accept established precedent. Even the most transformational improvements, once established, become the status quo.

Originally applied to manufacturing organizations, the concepts of Constraints Management have branched out successfully to many business environments, including service organizations, project-based companies, not-for-profits, and most recently, healthcare. By introducing Constraints Management, hospitals can gain significant insight into which areas to focus their performance-improvement efforts. In addition, there are many tools in the Constraints Management body of knowledge that can be used to improve flow, lead time, profits, return on investment, and project lead time, as well as to reduce inventory and operating expenses.

Figure 1.6 shows a process flow for inpatient procedures at a local community hospital. By mapping out the process flow and going through step one of the five focusing steps, the system constraint clearly can be identified to be housekeeping as it prepares the bed for the next patient. Although other steps in the process have significantly more capacity than nine patients per day, the real capacity of this process is determined by the capacity of the constraint, which is only nine patients per day. In fact, allowing any step in this process other than housekeeping to run at full capacity will result in suboptimization and patient dissatisfaction as patients wait endlessly for the housekeeping staff to prepare the next bed.

In steps two and three of the five focusing steps, our integrated approach deploys Lean and Six Sigma tools to increase the capacity of the constraint through process improvement by revealing the hidden capacity of doctors, nurses, beds, and operating rooms and by making sure that other steps in the process do not go faster than the constraint. If the demand on the process was still greater than the capacity of the constraint, then proceeding to step four, elevate, would be considered. This would entail adding additional resources—in this case, hiring more housekeepers.

Although a simplistic example, ask yourself how many times you have attempted to improve a step in a process that was more than likely a nonbottleneck step. Did the capacity of the entire process improve? This is the heart of suboptimization, and it is supported by many metrics that are used to measure processes that are centered on improving the output of each and every step in the process. Measurements such as capacity utilization and cost per process step encourage local optimization at the expense of the whole system. Constraints Management challenges these types of metrics and introduces a new set of metrics designed to ensure that

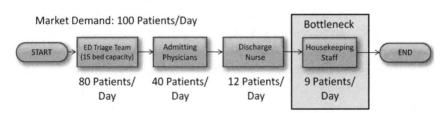

Figure 1.6 Process flow for a sample hospital.

holistic decisions are made. These use a technique called *throughput decision support*, which is described in more detail in Chapter 2.

The goal of steps one, two, and three is to get the most out of existing resources without spending additional money. Frequently these steps alone result in process improvement and the revelation of enough increased free capacity that incurring additional expense isn't necessary, and step four can be skipped entirely.

For example, suppose that a hospital's accounts receivable process is always delayed. By applying the five focusing steps, the constraint in that process is discovered to be the Coding Department. With the help of a *current reality tree*, root causes of payment delays are identified as errors within the Coding Department. By applying Lean and Six Sigma tools, three solutions arise, which include

▲ Establishing operational definitions for codes and procedures
▲ Developing coding lists with insurance companies
▲ Refining processes for the proper coding of procedures

As a result, coding errors become minimized, and the Coding Department is no longer the constraint in the accounts receivable process. The normal progression of the five focusing steps to step four is no longer necessary and can be bypassed by proceeding to step five and verifying that the hospital has sufficient capacity to satisfy the output of its accounts receivable process required by customers.

The power of Constraints Management is its ability to focus improvement efforts on the system constraints, preventing suboptimization and maximizing throughput. The five focusing steps, as well as much more about Constraints Management, will be examined more deeply in Chapter 2.

Conclusion

Healthcare faces shrinking budgets and decreasing reimbursements at an unprecedented scale. An aging population with ever-increasing demand for care—in both quality and quantity—will further exacerbate these issues. This is especially true in the United States, where more than 32 million people are expected to become insured because of healthcare reform. Outcomes need to be improved. Capacity needs to be increased. Costs need to be contained. Cost cutting, denying treatment, and meeting standards rather than pursuing excellence cannot possibly address these colossal challenges.

Transforming healthcare will not be accomplished overnight. The problems in healthcare have evolved over many years. While solutions may not be apparent today, what should be apparent is that the same approach that has been applied in the past is not the best way of moving forward. What also should be evident is that the more tools one has and the better the tools are applied, the better are the outcomes. You can use a screwdriver to open a can, but it will be difficult and messy. Integrated methodologies result in breakthrough solutions, which can be realized only through synergy rather than the application of a single methodology—out of the box and through three windows. The integrated approach allows it to be about the patient *and* the money.

Imbued throughout the integrated approach is an ability to get past the noise of competing objectives in order to concentrate on where it matters most. The philosophy, tools, and applications of Constraints Management exemplify this concept and can be found next in Chapter 2.

Constraints Management Applications in Healthcare

"Either you manage your constraints or they manage you."
—CHRIS ZEPHRO, CONSTRAINTS MANAGEMENT EXPERT

Throughout popular discourse, little has been publicized about Constraints Management applications in service industries, especially in healthcare. Since there is much information published about the application of Lean and Six Sigma in healthcare, in Chapter 1 their descriptions were kept relatively brief. On the other hand, Constraints Management applications in the medical field and related publications have been quite slow to gain recognition, particularly in the United States. This chapter will detail the evolution of Constraints Management, adapt its terminology to the healthcare environment, and elaborate on its applications: thinking processes, buffer management and supply-chain logistics, critical chain project management, and finance and measures.

The Evolution of Constraints Management

Constraints Management emerged as a management discipline more than 25 years ago, and since then, hundreds of success stories have been published about its application in the manufacturing industry. While the adoption of Constraints Management into service industries has been evident, it has not been as rapid nor as visible as it had been in manufacturing. Yet Constraints Management is now applied in distribution, engineering, hospital design, prisons, government, banks, software development, finance, legal services, cell phone companies, retail, education, insurance, marketing, sales, strategy, and change management, as well as various other services and enterprises.

The body of knowledge for Constraints Management applications has evolved, expanding in depth and breadth significantly since its inception. These applications, with examples from healthcare, will be summarized under four categories: thinking processes, critical chain project management, supply-chain solutions, and finance and measures. But first it might be helpful to review some early applications of Constraints Management in healthcare to introduce its terminology more generally.

Early Applications

The first healthcare application of Constraints Management that we are aware of dates back to 1991 in South Africa. It was pioneered in an outpatient department by Dr. Antoine van Gelder, who is a professor of medicine at the University of Pretoria Medical School and head of the Department of Internal Medicine at the Pretoria Academic Hospital. As detailed in the 2004 edition of *The Goal*, Dr. Gelder applied the buffer management solution, which in just six month's time reduced the department's waiting list from about eight months to less than four months. In another application at a 600-bed private hospital, Dr. Gelder's use of Constraints Management enabled a transition from a 20 percent budget shortfall to a profitable operation within a year. Despite these successes, very few applications in healthcare were reported until quite recently.

One of the earliest reported applications of Constraints Management in U.S. healthcare was at the University of Michigan Hospital. The hospital's admission and discharge system was inefficient, resulting in an average of three hours' delay in accepting incoming patients, who waited for their rooms to be prepared. Constraints Management allowed the hospital to reduce the average time to admit patients from 3 hours to just 11 minutes. According to an article by Jaideep Motwani and colleagues, the key to the hospital's success was better scheduling of housekeepers, cleaning dismissed patients' rooms by using beepers.

The 366th Medical Group of the U.S. Air Force at Mountain Home Air Force Base in Idaho was another team that applied Constraints Management logistic techniques successfully to "significantly reduce the time a patient waited between requesting an appointment and when the appointment actually occurred." The results of the team's work were reported in an article in *Journal of Healthcare Management* by David Womack and Steve Flowers. Using a two-pronged approach, the 366th Medical Group directed the five focusing steps on the processes of appointment scheduling and patient-provider encounters. The constraint identified in the appointment scheduling process was the availability of routine appointments. This constraint was exploited by replacing a fixed scheduling template with a dynamic appointment template, which allowed flexibility and no longer ignored variability of demand in the mix of appointment types.

The dynamic appointment template did not require radical technological innovation. It was simply a number of fixed scheduling appointment options for the following day. Each evening, the scheduler selected which appointment schedule template to use based on the demand seen throughout the day. By spending approximately 15 minutes per day, the appointment manager was able to "allocate provider time to patient demand," adjusting the schedule over the next day, week, and month to subordinate to the constraint of keeping routine appointment slots open. In refraining from allocating appointment slots dedicated for specific appointment types, much bottleneck capacity was freed.

Although it was assumed that the most expensive resource, the health providers, would be the bottleneck in the patient-provider encounter process, it actually turned out to be medical technician support. The team decided that shifting the constraint to the providers would be the most appropriate resolution on a long-term basis. The constraint was elevated subsequently when the team appropriated technicians from elsewhere within the medical group to improve the patient-provider encounter process, where they were needed to increase its capacity.

Between the improvements to the appointment scheduling and patient-provider encounter processes, the 366th Medical Group was able to achieve

▲ An approximately threefold decrease in routine appointment wait time from a preintervention high of 24 days to a sustained average of below the targeted wait time of 7 days

▲ A reduction in the average patient wait from 8 minutes to just 3 minutes, a 63 percent improvement

▲ Realization of these accomplishments at a cost of less than $200,000 and while freeing enough capacity to cover 800 more people, which was expected to generate over $1.6 million additional revenue

More recently Constraints Management applications seem to be flourishing among National Health System (NHS) hospitals in the United Kingdom. These NHS hospitals include University Hospitals in Coventry and Warwickshire, Derby Hospitals, Cardiff and Vale, Tauton and Somerset, Horton, Oxford Radcliffe, Oxfordshire, Frimley Park Hospital, Barnet and Chase Farm Hospitals, and Musgrove Park Hospital. Applications of Constraints Management also have been notably spreading across Dutch hospitals, including Maasstad Ziekenhuis, a health system consisting of two sites in Rotterdam with 600 beds, St. Maartenskliniek, and four more hospitals. Some of their success stories are summarized below.

Constraints Management Terminology for Healthcare

Since Constraints Management originated in manufacturing, its terms were conceived and defined originally in the context of production. Adapting Constraints Management for use by healthcare organizations does not require translation akin to learning a new language. It only asks us to expand our understanding of words we already know and to use them in a different way than we ordinarily use them. Fortunately, one does not need to understand everything about Constraints Management to be able to use parts of it almost immediately. Its most basic terminology can be attained from the following concepts: systems thinking, the goal, Throughput, constraints and their types, and the five focusing steps of Constraints Management.

Systems Thinking

Organizations are systems. Even a sole proprietorship consists of a single human body, which also could be described as a system. But just as a sole proprietor interacts with others throughout his or her dealings, be they with customers or with contracted associates, organizations interrelate with one another, and systems influence other systems. In fact, the definition of a system depends on where one is looking, and it is defined by its scope. Once a perspective is expanded beyond an immediate system, it becomes apparent that all systems are subsystems of larger systems. One could expand infinitely depending on how a system is defined.

Systems and processes are not synonymous, but they are interrelated. Within the scope of a process, there can be defined a system of interrelated components and variables. And every system includes one or more interdependent processes and incorporates interdependency internally, as shown in Figure 2.1. It is all a matter of perspective. The greater system of the universe, reality, or consciousness can be drilled down into the atomic process-level. The ability to change perspectives and understand the global, system-level impact of local behavior is the essence of systems thinking.

Constraints Management embodies a humanistic philosophy, much like the work of W. Edwards Deming, which assumes that people intrinsically want to do a good job and that many problems are not caused by people but rather by imperfect processes and systems. Constraints Management is also humanistic in that it does not believe in layoffs or across-the-board cuts. Systems thinkers understand that cutting costs in every department penalizes the most efficient, lean departments most and necessarily has a negative impact on the constraint, jeopardizing Throughput.

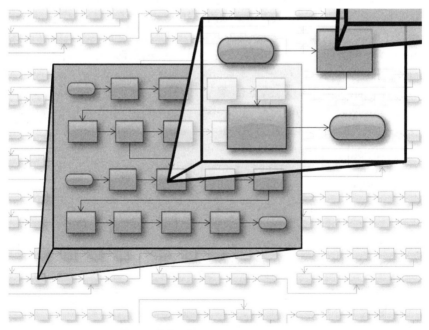

Figure 2.1 Systems and processes.

As an example, consider treatment of an advanced liver cancer patient using microsphere therapy. This therapy uses millions of tiny resin microspheres that contain a radioactive element. They deliver targeted internal irradiation therapy directly to the tumor. Using a small catheter, which is guided into the liver, microspheres are infused. The microspheres then are carried by the bloodstream directly to the cancerous tissue in the liver, where they deliver their dose of radiation. Figure 2.2 shows various systems and interdependent processes that need to function in unison and in a timely manner to provide this treatment successfully.

The actual treatment process cannot proceed unless the program director meets with the patient, examines the patient's history and current status, analyzes various imaging studies to determine whether the treatment is feasible from a medical perspective, and if feasible, prepares the treatment plan. The hospital needs to obtain insurance approval to schedule the procedure. The manufacturer of the microspheres needs advanced warning to custom manufacture the microspheres, which are produced overseas and require special shipment procedures owing to their radioactive content. Various dosimetry calculations and special approvals are necessary to place an order for the dose. Then the treatment needs to be scheduled by the Interventional Radiology Department, which is a shared resource. During various steps of the actual procedure, about 25 medical codes need to be entered correctly in order for the hospital to get reimbursed. In this specific case, nine different but interdependent processes needed to be analyzed.

If one were to draw the system boundary around just the treatment steps alone, suboptimization (i.e., not selecting the best value option from the organizational perspective) would be very likely. In summary, it is critical not only to look at the treatment process steps involving the patient in isolation but also to consider the entire system to increase Throughput. After all, even if the patient is not physically or directly involved, the quality of the treatment he or she receives nonetheless depends on the proper functioning of other elements in the system. If only the process perspective is considered, then system interactions may be missed.

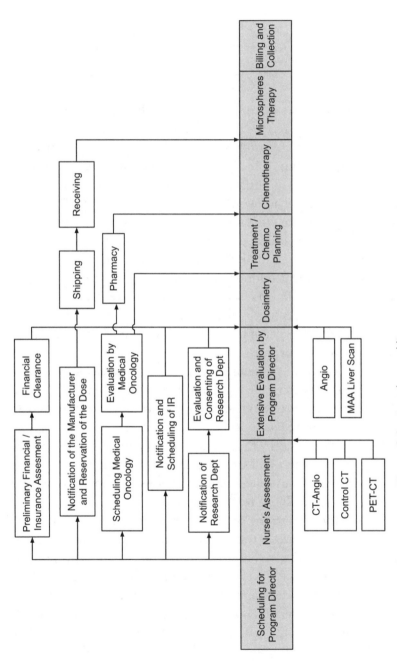

Figure 2.2 An advanced liver cancer treatment system.

The Goal

"Every system must have an aim; without an aim, there is no system."
—W. EDWARDS DEMING, FATHER OF TOTAL QUALITY MANAGEMENT

We have observed occasional confusion between the goal and the mission. A *mission* can be defined as the basic function of an enterprise or agency or any department of it. Another way of describing a mission is the business the organization is in. A mission may change, but goals rarely change. A goal is the end toward which activity is aimed—the end point of planning. If the mission is achieved, then what is the end result? The answer is *the goal*. The goal is the ultimate desired outcome for the system. Many hospitals have mission and vision statements, but only a few have goal statements that fit this definition. The prerequisites for any comprehensive Constraints Management solution are identification of the system's goal and critical success factors necessary to achieve that goal and determination of a means to measure goal attainment. Hence it is important to clarify the goal of the organization prior to implementation of Constraints Management.

The *TOCICO Dictionary* defines the *goal* as "the purpose for which the system was created as determined by the owners of the system." The owners of most for-profit companies identify the goal as "to make more money now and in the future," according to Goldratt. To achieve this goal successfully, they must satisfy their customers now and in the future, and they must provide a secure and satisfying environment for employees now and in the future. If customers and employees are not satisfied, the organization will be unable to reach the goal.

Within healthcare, a strong emphasis on making money is not widely embraced—and can seem contrary to the primary objective of healthcare, which is to provide care. While it is understood that the end result in healthcare is providing satisfactory care, care cannot be provided without financial viability. Financial viability therefore is a critical success factor to delivering care in the long run. Boaz Ronen has said that financial viability is like a hospital's health: Without it, the hospital has nothing. If it consistently runs over budget or its quality diminishes to the point that funding can no longer be acquired, financial viability has the potential to become the most critical issue a hospital faces. However, financial viability is "necessary but not sufficient," joining satisfied patients, employees, medical service contractors, and regulatory compliance as a critical success factor in many hospitals—even not-for-profits.

A variety of healthcare organizations exist, so it should not be a surprise if they do not share a common goal. Even within a given type, not-for-profit hospitals, for example, there is little agreement among organizations in choosing a specific goal. One way to resolve the question of defining such a goal is to realize that all not-for-profit service organizations share at least three critical success factors, without which the organization cannot reach its goal. All service organizations must keep its customers, employees, and shareholders satisfied. Without customer satisfaction, demand for services will cease sooner or later. Without satisfied employees, service delivery will be insufficient—either owing to a lack of capacity of resources or the tendency for unsatisfied employees to render service that customers find unsatisfactory. And if shareholder satisfaction is lacking, then financial viability and therefore existence can become compromised.

In their presentation at the TOCICO 2010 conference, Tom Shoemaker and Richard Reid encapsulated the three facets of satisfied shareholders, customers, and employees into an overarching goal applicable to all not-for-profit organizations: satisfied stakeholders, as shown in Figure 2.3. Although determination of value can vary greatly among stakeholder groups in a healthcare setting—most evident in the different perspectives between the payer and those receiving medical services—the concept of satisfied stakeholders usually resonates as the overarching goal.

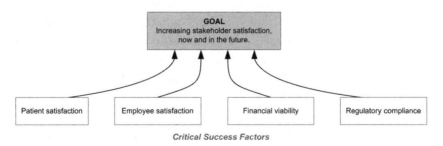

Figure 2.3 Critical success factors of a nonprofit hospital.

Throughput

Constraints Management emphasizes *increased Throughput* above all else as the primary means of improvement—even above cost-cutting activities—but not Throughput as it is traditionally defined. The traditional definition of Throughput, such as patient Throughput, refers to volume, or the rate of patients treated—patient volume divided by time. Besides the exception of financial viability and quantifiable clinical outcomes, value measurements in healthcare are commonly qualitative in nature. These qualitative measures include patient satisfaction and broad measures of regulatory compliance. Many metrics within healthcare do not capture the shades of gray of what actually occurs every day and must be force-fitted to be usable.

Constraints Management deviates from the traditional definition of Throughput. The *TOCICO Dictionary* defines *Throughput (T)* as "the rate at which the system generates *goal units*." Given Constraints Management's definition of a goal, applying units of measure to Throughput can better resonate in a healthcare setting if it were more easily measurable. Patient Throughput is closely correlated with financial Throughput, provided that the patient has insurance. In an emergency department setting, financial Throughput may be zero or even negative.

For healthcare, oral and maxillofacial surgeon and author Dr. Gary Wadhwa proposes treating the doctor as the constraint and the patient as the consumer, and he defines *Throughput* as the rate of cash generation through the delivery of high-quality, reliable service to patients. This means that Throughput is the payment for services related to a specific patient minus the totally variable cost of laboratory work, supplies, and so on for that patient. Wadhwa argues that any for-profit business must provide high-quality service to the customer and have satisfied employees as necessary conditions to stay in business. He adds that "making more money now and in the future," which is the goal of any for-profit business, is not possible without satisfying these two conditions. This definition can be acceptable for for-profit hospitals too. However, its applicability to not-for-profit hospitals usually creates passionate debate. Not-for-profit organizations cannot survive without strong cash flow to continue their day-to-day activities, and thus positive financial Throughput always must be maintained. It is a necessary condition.

Application of Constraints Management to not-for-profits is quite new, and there are different approaches about how to measure Throughput in these environments. Regardless of how Throughput is defined, throughout Constraints Management, one thing is consistent: When making decisions, increasing Throughput is always emphasized over reducing Inventory/Investment and Operating Expenses. More about Throughput and totally variable cost can be found later in this chapter under "Finance and Measures."

Constraints

In healthcare, a *constraint* is anything that impedes the ability or means to provide or deliver care. System constraints can be a resource, the market, or a supplier. In addition, they also can be a policy, artificial or permanent. The last three constraint types are not mutually exclusive with each other or the other constraint types, but they are useful designations nonetheless. Indeed, many resource and market constraints can be traced back to a policy that limits the organization's ability to produce more output, provide more services, or make additional sales. Policy constraints usually are difficult to identify but very easy to eliminate if management can see the cause-and-effect impact because they are entirely within management's purview. Resource constraints are relatively easy to identify and straightforward to manage and, if desired, eliminate. Many organizations strive to have no internal constraints and push their constraint into the market. Descriptions of these constraints are summarized below, but recall from Chapter 1 that the classification of constraint types is not yet standardized, and TOCICO is in the process of updating its dictionary.

Resource Constraints

A *resource constraint* (also referred to as a *physical constraint* or *bottleneck*) can be defined as any resource whose capacity is less than or equal to the demand placed on it during a specified time horizon, according to the *TOCICO Dictionary*. A resource constraint compromises the Throughput of the organization, effectively making it less capable of delivering service to meet the demand of the marketplace.

A resource constraint that commonly plagues hospitals is the lack of available space to treat and house patients. Constraints Management has been applied to the design of hospital layouts to optimize the flow of patients, doctors, and nurses to ensure that space does not become the constraining factor, according to a recent *Health Facilities Management* article by Frank Zilm. Resource constraint examples include

▲ Emergency Department (ED)—availability of ED physicians
▲ Operating Room—number of surgical cases per room or per day
▲ Anesthesiologists—ratio of number of operating rooms running to number of anesthesiologists
▲ Specialty clinics—availability of expensive technology (e.g., MRIs, PET scans)
▲ Labor and delivery unit—availability of birthing beds or monitoring devices
▲ Nursing—staff shortages during summer vacations and Christmas–New Years time off
▲ Doctors—scarce capacity of doctors within a private practice
▲ Fiscal—lack of capital budget

Market Constraints

A healthcare organization faces a *market constraint* if its capacity to provide its products or services exceeds patient or customer demand. The constraint in emergent-care scenarios preferably should be the market—a lack of patients who need emergency treatment.

A resource-constrained ED effectively means that if a patient presents with an emergency, he or she will be waiting for care owing to the fact that the resources he or she needs are not immediately available. It should go without saying that EDs are not the only part of healthcare organizations that should endeavor to operate at a high service level under a market constraint.

Market constraint examples include

▲ Multiple imaging service providers in the same geographic area offering similar services
▲ Dermatology capacity exceeding demand

Supplier Constraints

Supplier constraints, which can include material constraints, are frequently policy and/or resource constraints based outside organizational boundaries but within the organizational supply chain. They tend to arise because of problems subordinating or exploiting the supply chain's constraint owing to a focus on local optimization and poor planning. While a supplier traditionally may be defined as some entity outside an organizational system, Constraints Management duly considers the supplier because it is part of the "system" of the hospital. Suppliers are within an organization's span of control and sphere of influence such that it can choose other suppliers as well as bargain with them. And it is difficult to deny, especially in healthcare, that the lack of reliability of a supplier can be just as devastating to Throughput and patient outcomes as the lack of any other resource.

Supplier constraint examples include

▲ The provider of medication is unable to reliably fulfill orders in a timely manner.

▲ The lead time to receive an x-ray device is eight months when it is required now.

▲ Maintenance of an MRI machine is provided by the original equipment manufacturer as follows.

CASE STUDY

Supplier Constraint

A medium-sized hospital was experiencing a high failure rate of its MRI machine, and repairs of the equipment were outsourced to the original equipment manufacturer (OEM). Hence the repair process was controlled by the supplier. The repair contract gave the supplier up to seven days to repair the equipment. However, patients had to be rescheduled or turned away and sent to other imaging service providers when the MRI equipment failed. This resulted in lost revenue for the hospital as well as patient dissatisfaction. Since the hospital's demand exceeded the supplier's contractually defined capacity to repair the equipment, the supplier was the main constraint. However, a process value stream analysis with five focusing steps highlighted the opportunities to get the most out of the system. These included

▲ Frequent checks during the evening hours for service alerts

CASE STUDY

▲ Bringing duplicate spare parts for on-site repairs
▲ More preventive maintenance to avert failures in the first place
▲ Training on proper use of equipment and improving the diagnostics of malfunction
▲ Revision of financial approval policy eliminating red tape
▲ Streamlining of steps for repair to do it right the first time
▲ Strategic gating (defined later) based on patient types, making the best use of existing capacity
▲ Sharing failure data with the supplier to improve equipment design
▲ Renegotiation of the terms during contract renewal to improve response time and planned maintenance efficiency and effectiveness
▲ Reduction of handoffs to improve patient rescheduling and coordination, as shown in Figure 2.4

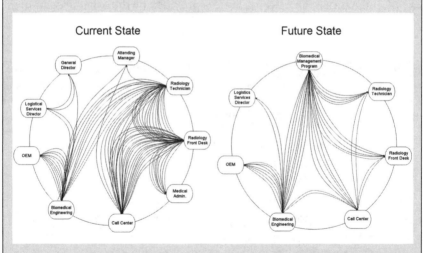

Figure 2.4 MRI repair and maintenance handoffs.

These actions allowed the hospital to make the most of its supplier; synchronize the related hospital resources and departments such as the call center, patient services, administration, and maintenance with its constraint; and thereby better manage it.

Policy Constraints

All the other constraints and almost any organizational issue having a significant impact on Throughput could be traced backed to or defined as a *policy constraint*. For example, level of staffing is a policy-level decision that immediately affects resource constraints. A policy might prohibit a hospital from accepting a certain type of medical insurance, which has a direct effect on a market constraint. Despite its overlap with other constraint categories, it can be useful to realize the unique characteristics of a policy constraint. Policy constraints have become evident by their observed prevalence throughout healthcare and other industries. There is no debate that bad policies can hinder the ability to get the most out of a system, so it is useful to recognize this fact.

Policy constraint examples include

▲ Hospital reimbursement according to length of stay, even if it is beyond the control of local leadership
▲ No overtime for any hospital staff (whether bottlenecks or not)
▲ Fixed number of patients for surgery per day
▲ No purchases of any kind between the twenty-fifth and month's end, including minor office supplies
▲ Payments based on procedures rather than outcomes

Artificial Constraints

An *artificial constraint* is synonymous with the term jointly coined by Boaz Ronen and Shimeon Pass, *dummy constraint*, as applied to resources. According to them, such a constraint exists when "the system bottleneck is a relatively cheap resource compared with other resources in the system" (reprinted with permission of John Wiley & Sons, Inc.). Expanding from this definition, an artificial constraint is a resource, market, supplier, or policy constraint that has no legitimate reason to be a constraint given its extremely low cost to break compared with the improved Throughput that could be reaped. An artificial market constraint may be a poor definition or segmentation of the population of potential patients. An artificial supplier constraint simply may be the selection of a less expensive but unreliable supplier when a better alternative is readily available, necessitating huge carrying costs owing to high safety stock levels. And a policy may be behind any of the aforementioned artificial constraints. The return-on-investment opportunity makes it overwhelmingly clear that anytime an artificial constraint is encountered, it should be broken. Artificial constraint examples include

▲ Reducing cleaning costs by hiring insufficient janitorial staff to clean and turn over operating rooms
▲ Operating rooms sitting idle owing to schedule conflicts
▲ Shortage of clerical staff to admit or discharge patients, procedures thus completed by physicians and RNs
▲ Scarcity of common hospital equipment, such as blood pressure cuffs, digital thermometers, and IV poles, creating backlogs in the ED and clinics

Permanent Constraints

Permanent constraints are not typical constraints in that they cannot be broken by elevation, that is, adding resources. Just because management attention is a permanent constraint does not mean that Constraints Management argues for an increase in midlevel managers; it argues for a change in the way managers approach management of the system. Permanent constraints are constraints in that they create inertia. While these are not *true* constraints in the strictest Constraints Management sense of the word, by changing how the system is addressed, managers can create new means to focus on the constraint and improve performance relative to the goal.

Since the complexity of organizations connotes interdependency, fewer independent chains exist, and thus there are fewer system constraints. One of the great strengths of Constraints Management is the clarifying focus it provides. It is important to bear in mind that while any of these four permanent constraints can act as the system constraint, by definition, the system constraint is *the* factor that *most* inhibits Throughput. Thus, while the resources of permanent constraints are expected to be fully utilized, managers still are advised to be mindful of the true system constraint and never lose sight of it.

Boaz Ronen has identified sales and marketing, information technology (IT), and research and development (R&D) as permanent constraints in organizations. In his keynote address at the TOCICO 2010 conference, Goldratt stated that he has become convinced that a constraint of any organization is management's attention. In healthcare, demand for IT, sales and marketing, R&D, and management attention frequently exceeds capacity—and by no small margin. Ronen has observed that expensive resources, such as dentists in private practices and anesthesiologists in hospitals, frequently tend to be permanent bottlenecks. Our findings throughout healthcare organizations have been concordant with these conclusions, so we have seen fit to describe the following permanent constraints.

Information Technology (IT)   Given that the processes by which organizations operate and direct information flows are never perfect and that the progress of technology is unceasing, improving IT to increase Throughput has unlimited promise. IT is inextricably entwined in business processes, so performance improvement likewise depends on it. This is the reason why practitioners map out not just physical flows of processes but also the flows of information within what Rummler calls "white spaces." In fact, there is an entire discipline, Business Process Management (BPM), resurging to address the divide among IT, process management, and improvement.

Technological change has become a goal unto itself, supplanting the true purpose of technology—to help the organization *reach* the goal. We have found too many processes that took a few steps with the technology of 20 years ago that now take many more steps with the modern technology of today. As a result, improperly implemented IT solutions waste the valuable time of doctors and nurses by introducing complexity, diverting time to serving the technology instead of caring for the patient. The prescription for this problem is to get away from handcuffing people with bad code and outsourced IT solutions, and to instead fix broken processes first before adopting technology.

Rushing to a boxed IT solution first usually means "more defects faster." Instead, IT personnel should be welcomed to participate in performance-improvement initiatives for not only their buy-in as critical stakeholders but also for their subject-matter expertise. With IT aboard, process improvement can happen concurrently with IT advancement in a union that benefits the entire organization. BPM, which evolved from Business Process Reengineering (BPR), has tools to be used within an integrated approach to performance improvement.

A chief information officer (CIO) of a hospital shared his views on IT within hospitals with us:

> There is a big disconnect among IT, medical doctors, and staff. It is important to eliminate this disconnect. These units need to understand each other from all aspects of the process. An IT

person is going to show resistance to a proposed change and work will be inefficient if the IT person does not clearly understand the process. If the hospital outsources, then the IT service representatives really need to know their craft so they can explain and control what is going to be done. By getting IT involved in Performance Improvement initiatives, projects will be completed faster and good results will be provided. Team members must keep in mind the resources of the organization and its preexisting technology infrastructure, and other IT constraints when determining the path taken in the long run. Finally, it should never be forgotten that IT systems are only as good as the data within them. Sloppy or haphazardly entered data does the patient a disservice: garbage in, garbage out.

In addition, a former CIO of a hospital stressed to us how critical it is to engage those who actually perform the work:

The best way to design processes is to ensure that the frontline staff are the main resources for analyzing the current process and designing the future refined process. These people often get overlooked and organizations miss a lot of great knowledge and insight and ultimately end up not having the best processes in place. I can speak to several automated health care processes that I have observed that had key input from people with nursing backgrounds, but they were not the nurses that perform that function on a daily basis. As a result, the processes that were designed are inefficient and fragmented because the key individuals were not engaged as the primary resources during the design stage. In short, the best people to design and build the process are those people that do it everyday.

To develop an IT solution without addressing and fixing existing process issues is the antithesis of technological advancement. Technological solutions should not create inertia and should be considered in novel, more relevant ways. Once bad code is adopted, it takes an inordinate amount of time to remove it because of the interdependency of other departments—especially IT resources, which are almost always overwhelmed and backlogged.

We have observed a number of improvement action items from value-stream analyses, rapid improvement workshops, and Six Sigma and Constraints Management projects that were delayed significantly or even completely owing to IT-related setbacks and interruptions. Whether it is identifying, exploiting, subordinating, or elevating a constraint, IT has a profound impact on to how to manage organizational constraints. The interdependency of people, technology, and processes within a given system should be made the most of in order to reach the goal. Technology should be a driver, enabling organizational success, rather than the reverse. It is a common practice for many organizations to try to force their staff into rigid off-the-shelf IT solutions. We often see how organizations make major IT investments without fixing their broken processes first and, as a result, do not realize significant benefits.

In the meantime, many process-improvement initiatives have IT-related action items, which usually take a very long time to complete. Thus an organization's internal IT capability can have a profound impact on performance-improvement initiatives, even affecting success. When a hospital determines its IT policy, it is making a fundamental decision that has an impact on the very foundation of the organization. Decisions regarding whether to develop code internally or outsource, select a particular software package, or agree to a specific maintenance and support contract should be made considering the system and the resulting inertia that a bad decision inevitably brings. IT is a permanent constraint, requiring collaboration, prioritization, and the investment of a *lot* of money.

There can never be a point in time when there is no better way that information systems could better manage data, including handoffs and coordination within healthcare organizations. Even if time stood still and technology did not advance, simply adding more technology may not help to achieve the goal. In order to improve the system, the way technology is applied must change.

Sales and Marketing Sales and marketing are considered permanent constraints because the market is potentially infinite and always can be redefined more broadly or narrowly so that demand for an organization's products and services increases. By further exploiting "the capacity" of its customers, the potential to realize more Throughput is infinite. For healthcare organizations, this means that treatments always can be spread further throughout communities. Growth in Throughput does not always portend more services or greater geographic coverage but rather services *more fit* to the population of potential patients or healthcare consumers.

Research and Development (R&D) As developed as a core competency can be, an organization always could do what it does *better*. Furthermore, there always exists the possibility of expanding into new areas of business because there are numerous ways to accomplish the mission and multiple missions to satisfy the goal, thereby achieving greater levels of Throughput. Put another way, the knowledge that could be learned about an organization's business always exceeds our capacity to grasp it all: There is always more that could be learned and researched. And as a result of research, better products and services could be developed forever. The service offerings of healthcare organizations therefore always could be expanded in scope and variety, and thus R&D is regarded as a permanent constraint.

Management Attention The constraint of any organization is management's attention, according to Goldratt. There are always more issues to increase Throughput beckoning for managers than they have time to work on. Even employees who feel that their bosses are micromanaging them freely admit that there are other, more pressing matters that their managers should be concentrating on instead. Fortunately, Constraints Management offers a rather unique remedy.

Recognizing that the way out of bad multitasking is not prioritization, the solution imbued throughout all Constraints Management applications is reduction of the number of tasks or orders that are open or outstanding, thus limiting or *choking* them. *Strategic gating*, or selecting the best projects to work on for the organization to reach its goal, allows managers to spend more of their time being productive rather than putting out fires. Strategic gating also entails *not* working on projects that do *not* help the organization reach its goal. Throughput decision support, discussed later, is an excellent tool that can be used to assist with strategic gating. Constraints Management does not advocate starting improvement by choking the release but rather examining whether improvements could be made "as is" without compromising Throughput. Buffer management itself, discussed later, also provides a mechanism to help managers allocate their attention.

The Five Focusing Steps

If there is a method characterizing the core of Constraints Management, it is the *five focusing steps*. These serve as a universal roadmap of sorts to achieve improvement in systems and thereby performance. As described in Chapter 1, the five focusing steps provide a simple, sequenced pathway not only to achieve gains but also to sustain them by avoiding inertia. Even an optimal solution deteriorates over time as the system's environment changes. A process of ongoing improvement (POOGI) is required to update and maintain the effectiveness of a solution—or replace it if it becomes outmoded or irrelevant.

Many organizations stop at step 3 because elevation in step 4 is not necessary depending on the constraint type and whether or not the capacity increase that resulted during the exploitation step was sufficient to meet the demand. Descriptions and examples of the five focusing steps applied to healthcare organizations are presented in Table 2.1.

Table 2.1 Focusing Steps of Constraints Management

Five Focusing Steps	Translation for Healthcare
1. *Identify* the system's constraint(s).	Identify the constraint at the system level: What most impedes the delivery of care? • Resource: Lack of nurses • Policy: Payer-network participation • Artificial: Nurses transporting patients • Market: Lack of patients • Supplier: Flu vaccine unavailability
2. Decide how to *exploit* the system's constraint(s).	Determine how to get the most out of the constraint: • Decrease the time it takes to prepare patients. • Shift portions of treatment to other resources with available capacity or where capacity could be added easily. • Modify treatment procedures to reveal hidden capacity. • Reduce the idle time of the constrained resource. • Operating rooms and other similar nonhuman resources do not need to take lunch breaks and can be scheduled to remain in use during such times.

(continued on next page)

Table 2.1 Focusing Steps of Constraints Management (continued)

Five Focusing Steps	Translation for Healthcare
	• A transporter does not abandon his or her post before a porter replacement arrives.
3. *Subordinate/synchronize* everything else to the above decision.	All elements of the system support the constraint via coordination and synchronization so that the bottleneck is never starved (assuming that the system constraint is a resource): • Purchase drugs and supplies based on demand and consumption. • Schedule patients based on doctors' capacity. • Stagger lunch breaks so that the phones of the call center are always answered.
4. *Elevate* the system's constraint(s).	Having completed exploit and subordinate, if the revealed/exposed capacity is insufficient, then additional capacity may be added, usually at some expense: • Buy an additional MRI scanner. • Hire more nurses. • Increase hours of operation. • Hire temporary workers for morning registration.
5. *Warning!!!!* If in the previous steps a constraint has been broken, go back to step 1 and do not allow *inertia* to become the system's constraint!	Be alert to adapt to changes in the operational, regulatory, and competitive environments, as well as changes to patient populations, because constraints can shift: • Healthcare reform • Accountable care organizations • Group purchasing organizations • If the system constraint changed, go back to step 1.

Applications of Constraints Management

There are many applications of Constraints Management. The following applications have been selected for discussion because of their relevance to healthcare, as well as their connection to the individual TOCICO certification categories. They are thinking processes for problem solving and strategy, buffer management and supply-chain logistics for service operations and logistics, critical chain project management for project management, and finance and measures. Table 2.2 shows typical results of Constraints Management applications.

Table 2.2 Constraints Management Applications and Typical Results

Thinking processes
Strategic planning, selecting high-impact projects, root-cause identification
Solution development
Conflict resolution with win-win
Breakthrough business performance improvement
Identification of high-reward projects
Accelerated project completion
Supply-chain and production
Managing constraints to maximize profits, reduce variation, optimize inventory
More than 50 percent reduction in inventory, order-to-delivery lead time
63 percent increase in Throughput/revenue
44 percent improvement in due-date performance
Finance and measures
Throughput decision support
Ensures making the right decisions from a financial perspective
Total alignment to maximizing the goal units
Ensures maximization of profitability at your given capacity
Critical chain project management
Project portfolio and single project management to accelerate completion
50 percent reduction in project duration
10 to 30 percent cost reduction
Stress reduction for employees, project managers, and senior leaders

Thinking Processes

"Nature is exceedingly simple and harmonious with itself."
—SIR ISAAC NEWTON, FATHER OF THE MODERN SCIENCE

Patients and physicians and payers, oh my! Healthcare, like no other endeavor, encompasses innumerable elements related in a multitude of complicated ways. To chronicle the sweeping variety of patients, ailments, treatments, departments, measurements, and payments would take more pages than are in this book. Complexity abounds in healthcare.

One of the fundamental tenets of Constraints Management is the inherent simplicity of all systems. In *The Choice*, Goldratt wrote, "The key for thinking like a true scientist is the acceptance that any real life situation, no matter how complex it initially looks, is actually, once understood, embarrassingly simple." Before learning how to read, words appeared to us as a garbled mess; before being taught how to tie our shoes, knots and bows seemed quite complicated. Constraints Management won't teach us how to read or how to tie our shoes, but its thinking processes can demonstrate how to do something almost as dramatic: It can teach us a different way of thinking, enabling us to solve the problems of complex organizations—even healthcare organizations.

By simplifying the complexities implicit in a healthcare organization, it becomes possible to discover the core drivers and not just outward symptoms. Rather than settling conflict with compromise, the thinking processes can defuse a conflict by exposing and rewiring the mistaken assumptions that trigger it, rendering it inert. A methodology that can reveal the source of any organization's problems and neutralize any conflict is especially relevant in healthcare. These are just two of the many capabilities that the thinking processes offer.

Predicated on the belief that people have immensely powerful intuitive faculties and are only lacking the discipline to harness their intuition's potential, the thinking processes provide a structured approach to problem solving with visual, logical maps. One need not have the logical prowess of Socrates to use the thinking processes, just some common sense and the will to exercise it. As Khaw Choon Ean detailed at her TOCICO 2006 conference presentation, the techniques and the reasoning are so straightforward and universal that young children all around the world have been taught to resolve conflicts successfully using the thinking processes.

The thinking processes are applicable in any problem-solving situation and do not require special adaptation for use in services. In published cases of Constraints Management adoption in services, a common approach is to start with the thinking processes and then use them to figure out which Constraints Management applications from industry might apply.

When used together, the thinking processes can answer the three basic questions related to change that Goldratt wrote about in *The Goal*:

▲ What to change?
▲ What to change to?
▲ How to cause the change?

These questions encapsulate what problem to focus on, what the solution is, and how to implement it. The original thinking processes approach begins answering the question, "What to change?" by building a *current reality tree* (CRT) to map the current state of an organization's problems and the conditions supporting them. The first step in creating a CRT is to generate a list of an organization's pain points, which can be obtained through a facilitated brainstorming session, but often such gripes, grievances, and grumbles are well known. They are the problems keeping managers up at night. Each problem is called an *undesirable effect* (UDE) owing to the interdependent nature of systems and the realization that each effect is the cause of other immediate effects; every consequence has an antecedent cause, which can be traced back *ad infinitum*. In other words, whether something is considered a cause or an effect is all a matter of perspective.

Treating manifested problems as effects of a deeper problem whose root cause is as yet unknown fosters restraint in rushing to judgment about a problem's underlying cause before appropriate analysis has been performed. In so doing, the label "undesirable effect" also encourages a systematic perspective by shifting emphasis away from fixing immediate superficial symptoms only to have what seemed like low-hanging fruit return again later. By using cause-effect-cause logical reasoning, UDEs can be linked together, and a CRT can uncover an organization's constraint or leverage point that most inhibits it from reaching its goal. A CRT also can reveal an organization's *core problem*, which the *TOCICO Dictionary* defines as "a fact, or conflict, or erroneous assumption that is the source of at least 70 percent of the undesirable effects in the current reality of the system being studied." We do not hold fast to a strict 70 percent definition and find that a "major source" and "large majority" of UDEs work as acceptable definitions, too.

Once the core problem on which to focus been identified, the next question to answer is "What to change to?" to begin to find a solution. A *conflict cloud* [also referred to as a *conflict resolution diagram* or an *evaporating cloud* (EC)] is a representation of a conflict illustrating the disagreement between the opposing sides in satisfying different conditions necessary to reach a common goal. For example, to satisfy the healthcare needs of a community, a hospital must both provide excellent healthcare service and control the size of its operating budget. The need to provide excellent quality care drives up spending on treating patients, whereas the need to control the size of the budget leads the hospital to reduce the amount of money spent on treating patients. What makes the conflict cloud such a powerful tool is that it facilitates the discovery of hidden assumptions that are invalid or can be invalidated by some future action, called an *injection*, that forms the basis of successful problem resolution. To continue to answer the questions, "What to change to?" and "How to cause the change?" other thinking processes tools are applied as described below.

When Goldratt and colleagues developed the tools of thinking processes from 1987 to 1992, they based them on two types of logical reasoning: sufficient cause (effect-cause-effect) logic and necessary condition logic. A piece of paper may be necessary to write a letter, but it is not sufficient because a pen or pencil also is needed. Based on this kind of reasoning, they created a set of five logical trees, or causal maps, as shown in Figure 2.5. Categories of legitimate reservation were developed to add rigor to the logical reasoning displayed in these trees, and they encompass the method by which the thinking processes approach is able to provide valid and reliable results. The tools were designed originally to function in concert with one another and are interrelated in that the output from one map is used as input to one or more other maps. However, they have evolved to a point where each can be used as an independent tool. According to a literature review in the *Theory*

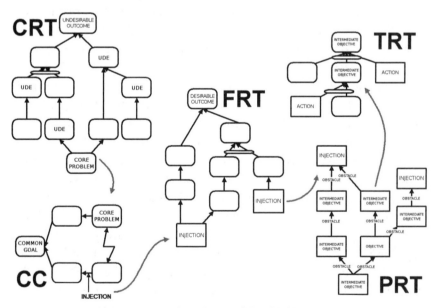

Figure 2.5 Original roadmap of the thinking processes.

of Constraints Handbook, about 41 percent of the time thinking processes are applied, it is the conflict cloud as a stand-alone tool.

Since their popularization in 1994 in Goldratt's book, *It's Not Luck,* it is not just the techniques themselves that have been evolving, there also has been an evolution in how they are applied. Rather than detailing various approaches, a short description of some tools and recommendations on ways in which to apply them based on our experience are provided. We have found the Intermediate Objectives map popularized by Dettmer and the focused current tree introduced by Ronen beneficial and a complement to the suite of original thinking processes tools such as the CRT and the conflict cloud. We highly recommend the Intermediate Objectives (IO) map for any healthcare organization facing a strategic gap issue. We also recommend application of a focused current reality tree (fCRT) when there is insufficient time to conduct a detailed CRT analysis. Even if a detailed CRT has been done, a simplified version of the CRT, called a *communication current reality* tree, should be developed so that the buy-in of individual executives, board members, and other stakeholders can be obtained. Communication CRTs are useful because they can be simplified for specific individuals. These trees allow individuals to appreciate their role in improving the system but not be overwhelmed by unnecessary detail. Chapters 3 and 6 describe how we make use of these tools. The suggested use of these specific techniques is not to the exclusion of the others, nor does it mean that other thinking processes tools are not as beneficial. We merely observed the challenges to implementation of the complete toolset in the often heavily resource-constrained environment of hospitals.

Where each tree is used is shown in Table 2.3 and described briefly below.

▲ **Intermediate objectives (IO) map.** Originally developed for applications of thinking processes geared toward strategy development, this is a diagram depicting the relationship between the goal and critical success factors that are required to reach the goal. Beneath the critical success factors, there are usually two layers of necessary conditions that must be satisfied to achieve critical success factors. The IO map represents a unified vision of where the organization wants to go and what the requirements are to get there. Dettmer wrote in his book, *The Logical Thinking Process: A Systems Approach to Complex Problem Solving,* that the IO map differentiates the discrete activities and outcomes to achieve the system goal and can help to build consensus

Table 2.3 Thinking Process Tool Utilization

Critical Questions	Step in Process	Technique
What is the strategic gap?	Determine the gaps to goal attainment.	Intermediate Objectives (IO) Map
What to change?	Identify the problem.	Focused Current Reality Tree (fCRT) Current Reality Tree (CRT)
What to change to?	Formulate the problem. Construct the solution.	Conflict Cloud (CC) Future Reality Tree (FRT)
How to cause the change?	Identify required actions. Action plan Implementation	Prerequisite Tree (PRT) Transition Tree (TT)

among the key stakeholders to support each other in a coordinated way. An IO map focuses the attention on which critical success factors are not yet achieved in order to identify high-level UDEs.

An IO map is a necessity-based logic diagram that facilitates answering the question, "What is the strategic gap?" As a logical extension of the prerequisites for the five focusing steps of Constraints Management, we ask this question before the three questions related to change established by Goldratt. We supplement the three original questions to establish the system and the goal of the system.

For an example of an IO map for not-for-profit hospitals, please see Figure 2.3 earlier. For more about using an IO map in the assessment phase of a performance-improvement deployment, see Chapter 4, including Figure 4.13, an example of an IO map for an outpatient service.

▲ **Current reality tree (CRT).** A CRT is a diagram that illustrates the cause-effect relationships that exist between the core problem and most, if not all, of the undesirable effects (UDEs). A CRT is a sufficiency-based logic diagram that facilitates answering the question, "What to change?"

▲ **Focused current reality tree (fCRT).** An fCRT is a "graphic managerial tool for helping to identify the core problems of the system or organization," as defined by Ronen and colleagues in the book, *Focused Operations Management for Health Services Organizations.* (Reprinted with permission of John Wiley & Sons, Inc.)

▲ **Conflict cloud (CC).** A CC describes and helps to resolve conflicts in a win-win manner as a structured method to facilitate the description and resolution of a conflict. Conflict resolution is accomplished via an injection, an improvement action necessary to reach a state where the conflict is resolved and erroneous assumptions are invalidated. A CC is a necessity-based logic diagram that facilitates answering the question, "What to change to?"

▲ **Future reality tree (FRT).** An FRT presents a sequence of cause-effect relationships that links injection(s) to their desired effects (DEs), the opposite of UDEs. Whether the injections come from conflict clouds or elsewhere, an FRT is a sufficiency-based logic diagram that facilitates answering the question, "What to change to?"

▲ **Prerequisite tree (PRT).** A PRT shows the relationship between the injections, intermediate objectives, and obstacles that block implementation of the injections. Intermediate objectives required to overcome the obstacles are included, and the sequence in which they must be achieved for successful implementation is shown. Rotated 90 degrees, a PRT is easily adapted to becoming a network node diagram for an improvement project. A PRT is a necessity-based logic diagram that facilitates answering the question, "How to cause the change?"

▲ **Transition tree (TrT).** Although use of TrTs appears to be diminishing of late with the preponderance of other tools, they are used for creating actionable plans for the implementation of solutions. It is a sufficiency-based logic diagram that facilitates answering the question, "How to cause the change?"

In a logical extension of these tools, several authors have begun experimenting with their use for analyzing and formulating strategy. In response, the *strategy and tactics (S&T) tree*, a graphic depiction of the hierarchal structure between goals, strategies and tactics, has emerged recently. This development was recognized at the TOCICO 2007 conference and again at the TOCICO 2010 conference when Goldratt attributed strategy and tactic trees with much of the success of maintaining continuous improvement in holistic implementations of Constraints Management in organizations in recent years. Goldratt described strategy as the answer to the question, "What for?" and tactics as the answer to the question, "How?" Linking tactics with strategy throughout healthcare organizations can ensure that all treatments, procedures, and operations are in alignment to the benefit of the patient. Although S&T trees are relatively new, their application to healthcare shows promise, as found in some early cases, such as Dr. Gary Wadwa's application of S&T trees in a dental practice.

In an environment as complex as healthcare, performance-improvement project selection is critical. In a performance-improvement deployment in healthcare, focusing on projects with a system-level impact will bring an organization closer to its goal and get more return from that initiative than a project with just a local impact. The tools of the thinking processes offer a robust solution to this project-selection issue, among others. Because they exemplify change, each thinking processes tool serves not only as a visual, logical gap analysis but also as a communication tool to overcome resistance and elicit buy-in from various stakeholder groups, according to the *TOCICO Dictionary*. A major contribution of thinking processes is their ability to unveil how certain policies and measures result in undesirable effects. With clear visual and logically sound depictions of the impact that bad policies have, it becomes easier to convince decision makers to break those policy constraints.

When an organization's culture lacks existing data and it is cost prohibitive to collect such data, such as destructive lot testing of pharmaceuticals for quality control, or data cannot be collected, the thinking processes are well suited for use. If, on the other hand, a culture of data has already been instilled, or if managers prefer a more quantitative than qualitative approach to performance improvement, designation of a Six Sigma project may remain a better option for the healthcare organization to pursue. On the other hand, thinking processes tools fit quite well inside a Six Sigma study too, as Chris Zephro pioneered at Seagate Technology and will be discussed further in Chapter 6.

The application of constraints management may result in unprecedented success for a healthcare organization. For example, in one case study cited by Julie Wright in her chapter on applications at large-scale healthcare systems in *Theory of Constraints Handbook*, it was reported that thinking processes helped a large hospital system triple patient Throughput with only a 5 percent increase in resources. If this result were not impressive enough, during the same period of time, the hospital system also sustained an increase in service quality of over 96 percent as well as in patient satisfaction of over 96 percent. Wright also cites that the thinking processes were instrumental in increasing the system's third-year operating profit margin to match the revenue of the entire first year of the hospital system.

In sum, the thinking processes use effect-cause-effect and necessary condition logic to identify core issues, leverage points, and conflicts in an organization; break the conflicts; and address systematic problems to reach the goal. As a problem-solving toolset, it is useful on its own within the context of a rapid improvement workshop or within a DMAIC project. However, when the thinking processes toolset is applied comprehensively in an organization, change is focused on where it will have the greatest benefit to the entire system, and without compromise, win-win breakthroughs become possible on a continuing basis.

Buffer Management and Supply-Chain Logistics

"A system of local optimums is not an optimum system at all."
—ELIYAHU M. GOLDRATT, AUTHOR OF THE GOAL

Having originated in the manufacturing environment, one of the most touted tools within Constraints Management is its supply-chain logistics solution, which incorporates buffer management. By understanding the interactions among resources, processes, and systems, managers can use the logistics tools of Constraints Management, such as drum-buffer-rope, buffer management, and replenishment, as not only a scheduling mechanism but also a means for improvement of the delivery of services throughout healthcare organizations.

Basics of Buffer Management

A buffer isn't just an appliance to keep floors looking shiny. Within conventional management paradigms, the most common type of buffer is safety stock—extra inventory kept on hand to prevent stock-outs, ensuring that products are available when customers demand them. The reason healthcare organizations are willing to incur the significant downsides of tying up capital, allocating storage space, and risking the expiration, perishability, and obsolescence associated with keeping a reserve of spare inventory is that the cost of stock-out is huge—perhaps even immeasurable. But the real reason why safety stock is maintained is uncertainty: uncertainty owing to variability from both suppliers and customers. In a perfect world, where suppliers and transporters are always reliable and customer demand can be predicted with accuracy, there would be no need to keep safety stock. Although safety stock is just one type of a buffer, the true purpose of buffers generally is revealed by its example.

When anything is scheduled to occur literally just in time, unforeseen delays don't have the chance to hinder the timely completion of tasks—any interruption necessarily slows things down, by definition. When the operations of an entire system are scheduled to be just in time, the impact of a single delay isn't felt just locally; it has a ripple effect throughout the entire chain of subsequent tasks in the process. With such a timetable, the resources at any step have the potential to become overwhelmed. Scheduling all required materials, information, and inputs to arrive precisely just in time means that the unbridled impact of Murphy's law will be felt harshly without any safety. In Constraints Management, Murphy's law is affectionately known as *Murphy*, which is *special-cause variation*. It is not a question of *if* but a question of *when*. Simply put, scheduling logistics and other operations with just a little bit of buffer can improve flow. When things are scheduled to arrive just before they are needed instead of exactly when they are needed, a time buffer is introduced. Like safety stock, this buffer is helpful to control for variability and uncertainty.

In fact, by not scheduling anything except for the true process bottleneck, the rest of the process can be robust, flexing to accommodate natural variation. Instead of making each step of a process have just enough capacity, sprint capacity naturally exists, by definition, in all nonbottleneck resources. Rather than pursue the illusory ideal of a perfectly balanced line, Constraints Management recommends acceptance of the tendency for systems to have unbalanced capacity and leveraging existing capacity. The aim of Constraints Management is to balance flow rather than capacity. Besides, balancing capacity may be undesirable financially or practically. Sprint capacity is synonymous with protective capacity because this extra capability protects the Throughput of the system when Murphy strikes and even during periods of natural variation. Sprint/protective capacity, time cushions, and extra inventory all can act as buffers to safeguard against uncertainty. Constraints Management demonstrates how it is possible to use time buffers and sprint capacity to accomplish the same defense while reducing the need to hold excessive inventory.

Buffer management connotes several ideas, all stemming from using buffers as a way to manage. Besides introducing an interval that provides a bit of extra time to ensure that the bottleneck does not starve and that the system can complete its tasks on time, buffer management goes well beyond that. In addition to prioritizing work for the constraint on which to take action, buffer management provides the mechanism for continuous improvement and focused management. A prime place for processes to measure themselves is the buffer. Since service times are being collected and tracked in the same system that tracks time buffers, reasons for services being completed better than expected, as well as causes for why services are being delayed, also should be recorded so that they can be analyzed for improvement opportunities.

From a logistics perspective, it is key for healthcare organizations to have enough resources and to use them effectively so that patients move through health service processes smoothly, without interruption. As Julie Wright astutely points out in the *Theory of Constraints Handbook*, "The only factor that should impede a patient's progress through the caregivers' services should be the patient's ability to heal or recover, with no system- or clinician-imposed wait times"—the patient's body's ability to heal itself is indeed where the constraint ideally should reside in healthcare.

For example, on admission to several NHS hospitals in the United Kingdom, Stratton and Knight's buffer management application calls for calculation of a planned discharge date for an expected course of treatment or a given a treatment plan. It is against this buffered prediction that delays in patient flow are analyzed and optimized in order to discover what is problematic upstream and downstream in the process. Hybrid solutions that combine two types of Constraints Management scheduling systems, called *drum-buffer-rope* and *critical chain*, have been applied to treating patients as projects because, like projects, individuals and their health and treatment plans are unique and customizable. A green-yellow-red traffic light color coding system common to other buffer management applications, such as replenishment, is frequently employed. It is quite useful in directing the permanent constraint of management's attention within logistics operations.

Drum-Buffer-Rope

Drum-buffer-rope (DBR) is a mechanism to schedule the logistics of production in manufacturing settings, but it is just as applicable in services. The *drum* is the pace of the constraint, which governs the pace of the system. The *buffer* is the time a unit, patient, specimen, or diagnostic arrives at the constraint before it is scheduled to be worked on. The *rope* is the choked release of new units, raw materials, patients, or customers into a system to begin being worked on, as governed by the drum. In a DBR system, scheduling of all resources is not needed because only scheduling work done by the constraint is required.

DBR is implemented as a natural extension of the five focusing steps. Step one identifies the drum, step two identifies how best to place the buffers in order to exploit the drum, and step three subordinates the system to the drum by linking the constraint to the release of new materials and/or customers into the system. If this is not sufficient to achieve movement of the constraint from internal to external/market, then step four, elevation of the constraint, may be necessary if a sound business case can be made for adding additional capacity (Figure 2.6).

Simplified drum-buffer-rope (S-DBR), an adapted form of DBR, is appropriate to use when there is no internal constraint and the constraint is in the market. In hospitals using S-DBR, the patient demand becomes the drum. The key concept in S-DBR systems is subordination to the market, although key resources should continue to be monitored to ensure that the constraint has not moved back inside the system (Figure 2.7).

One of the keys to Constraints Management is to make sure that the bottleneck is never starved in a system. This is accomplished by using buffers at strategic locations. For example, at an ophthalmology clinic, a buffer system was set up to prevent wasting time between patients. Instead of calling patients one at a time, the clinic called two patients at a time to ensure that a surgeon never waited for a patient to be brought. The clinic

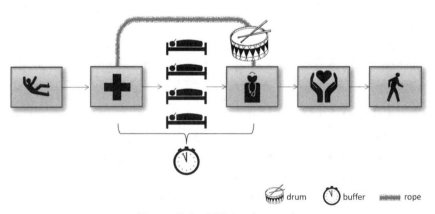

Figure 2.6   DBR in a hospital.

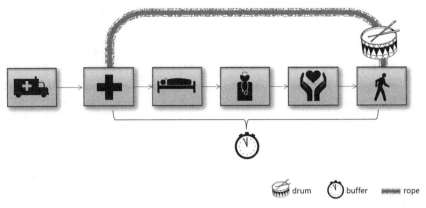

drum   buffer   rope

Figure 2.7   S-DBR in a hospital.

arranged a small room close to the operating room as a waiting area. Later, this buffer was unnecessary because the heightened attention of the staff subsequently resolved the issue of surgeons waiting for patients.

Numerous success stories were published about buffer management applications at hospitals in the United Kingdom. Alex Knight presented his impressive accomplishments throughout the NHS in various publications and conferences. Some of them are summarized below.

At the Accident and Emergency (A&E) Department of Oxfordshire Horton Hospital in the United Kingdom, personnel were able to process only 50 to 60 percent of the patients in less than 4 hours in 2002. In addition, the acute hospital admitting process frequently exceeded 4 hours, often surpassing the imposed 12-hour waiting period limit. The buffer management process was implemented in March 2003, and in five months, the percentage of A&E patients processed in less than 4 hours improved to 91 percent. Twelve-hour trolley waits were completely eliminated as well. Similar results were reported at Oxfordshire Radcliffe Hospital.

Cardiff and Vale NHS Trust, the third largest NHS member in the United Kingdom, implemented Constraints Management to discharge planning on 30 wards (10 acute, 10 mental health, and 10 rehabilitation). By estimating a predicated date of discharge (PDD) to set up managed buffers for each patient based on his or her expected course of treatment, the rendering of medical services was expedited when the expectation of a timely discharge became jeopardized. Buffer management, promoting clear visibility of patient status and length of stay in the healthcare system, is attributed with much of Cardiff and Vale NHS Trust's success: an 8.5 percent reduction in length of stay, a 50 percent reduction in health-related lost bed days, improvement against the A&E Department 12-hour targets, meeting elective waiting time targets, achieving financial balance, and reducing the wait for neurologic rehabilitation from several weeks to a few days.

According to Martine Price, director of governance and nursing at the Taunton and Somerset NHS Foundation Trust, Constraints Management was "applied to improve patient flow in A&E, assessment units, and discharge planning . . . [which] . . . has resulted in a sustained reduction in medical length of stay from 8.6 to 6.3 days (>25 percent)." The target in the United Kingdom is for NHS hospitals to treat 98 percent of all A&E Department patients within four hours, and Constraints Management's logistical solutions are helping the NHS to attain this service level. Barnet and Chase Farm Hospitals NHS Trust went "from one of the worst performing trusts in England to one of the top performing" when it became "the top performing trust in London for the four-hour target and 6th across England." Another NHS hospital was able to reduce its length of stay by up to 23 percent.

In 2000, Russ Kershaw reported in *Accounting Management Quarterly* that an outpatient oncology clinic experiencing growing demand used the five focusing steps of Constraints Management to increase treatment capacity from an "average 24 to 25 patients per day" to "an average of 30 patients per day," an improvement of 20 to 25 percent. By examining patient flow, the clinic's managers identified that the bottleneck resource was chemotherapy treatment chairs. To exploit the bottleneck, the clinic sought to minimize the time that patients occupied treatment chairs. Rather than registered nurses hunting for veins and providing posttreatment education while patients were seated in the treatment chairs, well-qualified lab technicians established intravenous access for most patients while they were at the lab for blood tests beforehand, and the RNs performed the posttreatment education during chemotherapy treatment instead of afterwards. The clinic was able to reduce the "average treatment time from 2.5 hours to about two hours," and its managers expect that once other leading consumers of bottleneck time are mitigated by "alternative procedures for initial treatment training and blood transfusions, . . . the clinic would be able to provide chemotherapy treatment to 35 to 40 patients per day, which represents a 40 to 67 percent increase in the clinic's treatment capacity."

Replenishment: Supply-Chain Problems at Hospitals

Emerging technology, shifting population demographics, governmental regulation, and skyrocketing costs have elevated the business of healthcare to an unprecedented level of global scrutiny. One of the primary drivers of the escalating cost of healthcare is the cost of materials management. Hospitals and health systems soon may spend more on their supply chains than on labor. Historically, total supply expenses have consumed up to 45 percent of a typical hospital's operating budget, and a recent analysis by Jamie C. Kowalski suggests that by the end of 2011, it could exceed 50 percent. While improvements to supply-chain management have been widely noted in the shipping, textile, big-box retail, and e-commerce industries, three factors have made it difficult to translate the advances achieved in other industries to healthcare: complexity, unpredictability, and risk.

In the United States, the healthcare supply chain involves more than 650,000 different manufacturers, distributors, carriers, Group Purchasing Organizations (GPOs), hospitals, clinics, and providers. A single ailment can involve multiple interdependent yet disparate entities: primary-care providers, specialists, pharmacies, diagnostic imaging and laboratories, outpatient surgical centers, hospital patient care units, anesthesiologists, surgeons, physical and occupational therapists, and others. Within the hospital, each department, area, and role has unique needs and multiple ways of obtaining supplies. A single patient care unit may use point of use, par level, perpetual inventory, case carts, requisitioning, and consignment. And physicians' preference of multiple types of supplies that could be standardized requires not only more storage space but also the additional management of codes and general ledger entries, making the system even more complex.

Linkages between clinical operations, materials management, and the supply chain, if they exist, are often fragmented and insufficient. There is no integrated, seamless flow of information from the bedside, where demand occurs, to the disposition, where capacity is established. Information must be translated manually from one system's format to another's, compounding wasted time, cost, and the potential for error at each exchange.

There is no way to estimate, with confidence, the number of patients and the vast variety of symptoms they present on any given day. This unpredictability has significant ramifications: The consequences of underestimating the appropriate inventory of a type of antivenom or artificial heart valve are far different from those associated with bicycle or computer parts. The potential consequences of stock-out include disability and even death, along with litigation. Nurses hoard supplies and patient care units maintain safety stock above par level because of the personal and professional risk involved. Until a system is developed that can consistently stock what is needed to care for patients before it is needed, providers will continue to resist efforts to cut supply costs. These competing goals result in the conflict expressed in Figure 2.8, an inventory conflict cloud.

The conflict involves the increasing versus decreasing inventory. Both positions have the common goal to increase financial viability, but the rationale and conclusions are different. The first argument states that in order to increase financial viability, we must protect supply availability, and in order to do that, we must increase inventory. The other side of the conflict argues that to increase financial viability, we must control cost, and the only way to control cost is to lower or limit the amount of inventory. The key to resolving the conflict is to focus on the impact of improved supply-chain management on patient care, not solely on product acquisition costs. A more efficient supply chain not only will add to the bottom line but also will reduce the time that healthcare workers spend on administrative tasks, allowing them to focus on delivering quality patient care. Perhaps most significantly, the increased availability of medical supplies when needed is a prerequisite to assuring the highest-quality patient care possible. Linking

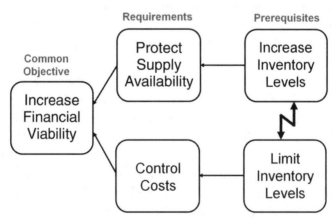

Figure 2.8 Inventory conflict cloud.

patient outcomes to value in a holistic collaboration that answers the question, "What's in it for my patient?" ("WIFMP?"), removes barriers to change, facilitating implementation and ensuring sustainment.

The Conventional Approach

In the conventional approach to supply-chain management, hospitals depend on forecasts of expected customer demand in what is called a *push system*. In a push system, a management decision must be made far in advance, at each reorder, regarding the amount of supplies to be purchased and how often to reorder. Inventory is pushed downstream through the links of the supply chain to reduce the appearance of excessive over-inventory, clogging the supply chain with inefficiency.

The problems associated with executing to forecast are

1. Stocking the wrong medicines, which can result in too much of one type of medicine and not enough of another
2. Limited responsiveness to true demand by patients and doctors
3. Pressure on cash flow
4. Inventory erosion, spoilage, and obsolescence
5. Inventory being pushed into the system, which results in loss of control, including hoarding

Conventional healthcare supply-chain management balances on the accuracy of forecasting. Forecasting should be used for what it was created for originally—*planning*. Most forecast problems arise because almost all organizations use it for planning *and* execution, and this is where the problems start. Missing the forecast is almost a 100 percent guaranteed result. If a forecast reads, "We will use 600 orthopedic joints for the month of June," this translates into an order for 600 orthopedic joints from a supplier. But the chances that the hospital will use exactly 600 joints in the month of June are extremely slim. At the end of the month, the hospital either will have excess orthopedic joints or will have stocked out before the month's end. Organizations need to accept the fact that forecasts are never correct and should be used for planning purposes only. It's much better to plan to within a reasonable range rather than a single-number forecast. Constraints Management expert Chris Zephro put it best when he said, "Plan to forecast and execute to demand."

The Solution: Dynamic Replenishment

The key difference between *dynamic replenishment* and conventional approaches is that it is fundamentally a *pull system* rather than a push system. A pull system controls the flow of supplies by automatically adjusting inventory levels based on actual consumption, with strategic buffers of inventory for each item to act as shock absorbers, compressing when inventory is consumed until replenishment occurs.

Each time an item is consumed, an equivalent order is placed. Replenishments occur in the smallest possible batches as frequently as possible. Thus statistical variations are dampened rather than magnified, reducing fluctuation of stock levels across the chain. In considering whether to adopt dynamic replenishment, because of the need for more frequent ordering or shipment, there may be some concern about transportation costs increasing. The easy way to justify the more frequent shipment of smaller quantities of a particular product is through the batching of orders for many products to achieve economic transportation quantities. The benefit of Dynamic Replenishment is not more frequent shipments but rather the receipt of the same number of shipments but of mixed products rather than frequent shipments of a single product. Figure 2.9 shows the more frequent replenishment cycles of a pull inventory system, which therefore is more responsive to the market and holds, on average, less inventory than a push inventory system.

Figure 2.10 depicts not only the traditional flow of materials in a hospital supply chain but also the flow of consumption information under

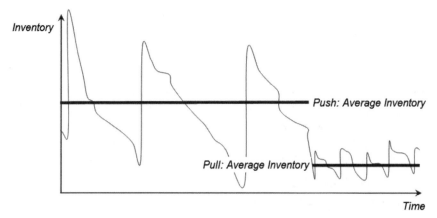

Figure 2.9 Push versus pull inventory replenishment systems.

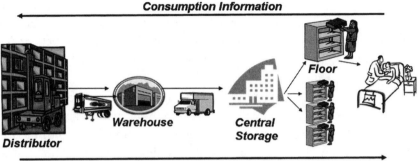

Figure 2.10 A hospital supply chain.

a dynamic replenishment system. This picture highlights the increased visibility that dynamic replenishment provides throughout the entire supply chain in terms of inventory levels and point-of-use demand.

Since supplies flow downstream, most of the inventory remains further up the supply chain. This reduces the amount of safety stock across the supply chain. Yet shortages are also reduced because of constant flow and rapid response to consumption. Buffer management matches stock of each product at each location to changes in replenishment time and demand, adjusting buffer sizes continuously.

One-to-one ordering with frequent replenishment, combined with buffer management, liberates hospitals that adopt pull from reliance on inaccurate and unreliable forecasts. Implementing a pull system increases revenues without increasing Operating Expenses and typically reduces investment in inventory. This improvement in Throughput is driven by increased availability and provides better-quality healthcare for the present level of cost or less.

The dynamic replenishment solution consists of four key components:

▲ Centralization of inventories
▲ Development of inventory targets based on replenishment time
▲ Absorption of variation in demand and supply by strategic buffers
▲ Synchronization of supply flow achieved through a focus on the status of inventory pulled into the system over time

For most organizations using push inventory systems, once product is pushed out into the channel, it is very difficult to move it to another location if that inventory is required somewhere else. This is typically due to IT system limitations, local hoarding of inventory, or most commonly, the cost associated with cross-shipping. Often sites requiring more products prefer simply to order more rather than to cross-ship, which results in increased total system inventory.

In the dynamic replenishment framework, a central warehouse is used to service regional warehouses and/or consumption points, giving organizations the ability to serve inventory to the locations that need it most based on actual consumption. Another benefit of establishing a central warehouse in the dynamic replenishment framework is to absorb demand variability. Variability in consumption is highest at consumption locations. By introducing a central warehouse that serves multiple locations, variability actually is reduced. Since the demand from a supply point is the aggregated consumption of all the points it feeds, statistical fluctuations average out. Thus, as the number of consumption points the central warehouse serves increases, the variability at the central warehouse decreases. Consolidation of inventory at a central warehouse allows reduction in the overall level of safety stock required to achieve the same or better service levels and availability.

By adopting a dynamic replenishment solution where inventory is pulled into the system by demand signals, the impact of incorrect forecasts is mitigated because the dependence on forecasting is diminished. With dynamic replenishment, inventory can reach an optimal level to meet a given service requirement. While every circumstance is unique, it is not uncommon for inventory carrying costs to decrease by 30 to 50 percent, or even more, while availability flourishes with no stock-outs. This availability is accomplished simply by replenishing more frequently based on what is consumed and strategic buffering. For example, an inventory analysis of selected medical supplies we conducted showed an inventory reduction potential of about 70 percent. Dynamic replenishment is not recommended solely as an inventory-reduction system. The improved inventory reduction is a one-time event. It is much better to promote the solution based on improved availability of inventory, which results in greater Throughput in the long term.

Dynamic replenishment also offers the added benefit to managers of leveraging their attention to focus on just the stock-keeping units (SKUs) where their intervention is needed. Dynamic replenishment and active monitoring not only foster a more responsive system but also alleviate risk by ensuring that medical supply levels are sufficient to meet patient demand without stock-out, thanks to increased ordering opportunities and directing management's attention to where it is needed most. Increasing inventory turns frees up operating cash that otherwise would be tied up in inventory while reducing obsolescence and spoilage. And drastically reducing inventory costs allows healthcare systems to spend those funds where it counts most—on improving patient care.

Critical Chain Project Management

"Focusing on everything is synonymous with not focusing on anything."

—ELIYAHU M. GOLDRATT, AUTHOR OF THE GOAL

Projects pervade healthcare systems. Whether one considers hospitals, clinics, laboratories, medical suppliers, or the pharmaceutical industry, the ability for healthcare organizations to manage projects successfully has become a necessity. Driven by such demands as improvement to the quality of patient care, compliance with new regulations, acceleration of the R&D process to bring new drugs to market faster, and other factors, it is little wonder that projects affecting healthcare are in such abundance.

Project management, the systematic way of planning and managing time and resources to achieve unique, finite goals, probably has existed in one form or another for at least 5,000 years. After all, the Egyptian pyramids and other great ancient structures did not just build themselves—they were carefully planned and managed. Ad hoc and calendar-based planning methods have been used throughout history, but it was not until 1917 that an easy-to-understand display, visually organizing tasks and time, was brought into the modern workplace—Henry L. Gantt's chart, now called the *Gantt chart.* Gantt charts were used in a multitude of projects, such as construction of the Hoover Dam (1931–1936) and the Manhattan Project (1942–1945).

The toolset of project management expanded when the critical-path method (CPM) was developed by DuPont in 1957 and the program evaluation and review technique (PERT) was developed by the Special Project Office of the Department of the Navy and Booz Allen Hamilton in 1958. Using CPM and PERT brought improvements over Gantt charts in the ability to manage projects with large numbers of tasks, interdependent tasks, and tasks with uncertain completion times. These methods were used to send people to the moon in the Apollo Program (1961–1972), as well as countless other projects since their advent. A timeline of project management methods appears in Figure 2.11.

As powerful as these tools have been, critical chain, a project management strategy and philosophy, represents the next major step in the progression of project management. Building on earlier advancements, critical chain cultivates the enhanced visual management and node networking aspects of its predecessors as well as incorporating new capabilities. While not diminishing the importance of other project management methodologies, professors of executive healthcare management, such as William Millhiser, of CUNY Baruch College, have noted that students frequently ask, "Why do you teach PERT when we learn so much from *critical chain?*" Identification and scheduling of project activities allow proactive management of variability. Critical chain can be of enormous utility in ensuring that healthcare projects are completed on time, within budget, and delivering all promised objectives. Instead of managing projects so that each task is completed on schedule, critical chain principles help to determine where to focus so that the entire project is done on time.

By strategically scheduling tasks and resources, critical chain positions flexible buffers at key leverage points in dynamically changing environments to absorb the shocks of unpredictable delays. By alerting relevant parties when projects begin to become delayed or when upcoming work will become crucial to the timely completion of projects, intervention can be well timed so that scarce management attention becomes focused where it will be most beneficial to the system.

Well-managed buffers can help not only to adapt to the normal variation that exists in projects but also to serve to highlight special causes of delays when they occur. In this way, critical chain introduces a feedback loop so that managers can better understand processes underlying projects and serves the

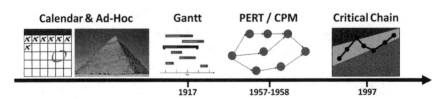

Figure 2.11 Project management methods timeline.

overall goal of developing a culture where performance improvement is practiced. Many medium-sized or large healthcare organizations are multi-project environments. Here, *pipelining* projects, or the strategic staggering of projects, becomes vital to resolving conflicts caused by contention for shared resources and makes adept use of a system's constraints.

And unlike conventional project management methods, critical chain combats many of the behavioral tendencies people have that delay projects, such as *bad multitasking*, the unplanned switching between unrelated activities. Multitasking is not unique to healthcare; in today's fast-paced business culture, most multitasking is regarded positively and even encouraged. However, suspending work on one task in order to work on another, unrelated task necessarily will delay completion of the suspended task. In such instances, multitasking becomes bad. This phenomenon is illustrated in Figure 2.12, which depicts the juggling of three tasks, A, B, and C.

By switching among tasks A, B, and C, each task finishes later than it would if the tasks had been done in sequence. The figure approximates the reality of the problem because delays caused by people forced to reorient

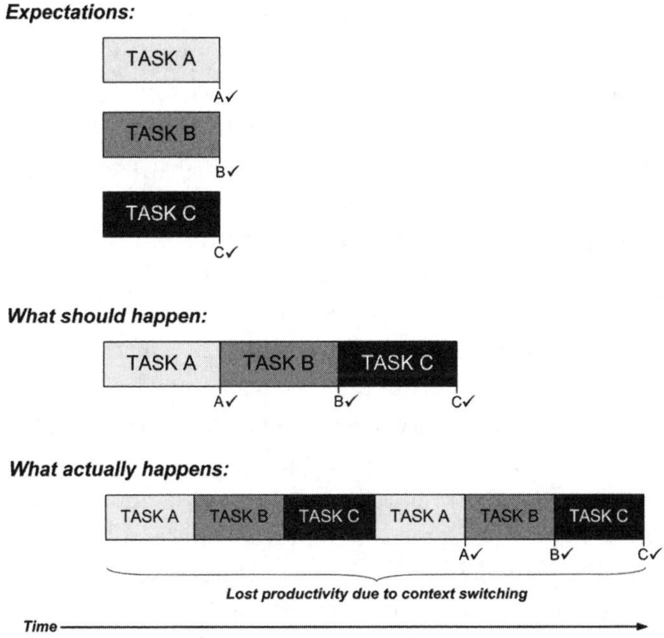

Figure 2.12 The impact of bad multitasking.

themselves on their return to work on dormant tasks are taken into account. One can consider how nurses are called away from direct patient care to work on other duties and then must redirect their attention back to the patient to better understand this experience. Moreover, when this switching delay occurs on certain critical tasks, the timely completion of entire projects can be compromised.

Beyond bad multitasking, critical chain is designed to mitigate other human tendencies that can cause projects to be late. Even otherwise responsible adults can exhibit *student syndrome* by procrastinating from starting work until just before it is due. *Parkinson's law* suggests that work expands to fill the time allotted for its completion, for example, continually polishing a report rather than assessing that it is good enough and moving onto other, more pressing matters. *Sandbagging*, or withholding the submission of completed assignments until they are due, is justified by some as a way to manage the boss's expectations and preventing future deadlines from encroaching.

Critical chain even provides a way to counteract the safety time people add to inflate their time estimates to ensure that they will be able to complete their assignments by their due dates. Promoting high work visibility and clear status tracking, critical chain methods foster team trust and a relay-runner work ethic, which allows projects to be completed with the same resources at a much faster rate—20 to 50 percent faster or more in many established implementations. All that are needed for critical chain's implementation are commitment from management, honest communications, strategic planning, and buffer management. Tools and technology can help people in prioritizing and scheduling their time to act in accordance with the success of projects and, ultimately, the organization's objectives (Figure 2.13).

Project management success stories using critical chain have been reported widely in varying industries by such companies as Boeing, Hewlett-Packard, and others. After having used it in 2,523 public works projects in 2007 and over 4,000 public works projects in 2008, the Japanese government has recommended that critical chain project management (CCPM) "be used on all projects henceforth (approximately 20,000 projects per year)." The widespread use of CCPM resulted in average project durations cut by 20 to 30 percent or more, with some companies able to complete twice as many projects in the same timeframe with the same resources.

Critical chain has proven its suitability and success for projects in the healthcare industry. In early 2008, Maasstad Ziekenhuis, a Dutch health

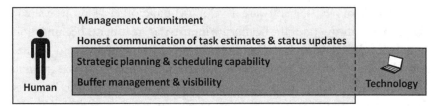

Figure 2.13 Requirements for critical chain.

system consisting of two sites in Rotterdam with 600 beds, was expanding to open a new hospital and reportedly had 180 open projects in its pipeline. Beyond the design and construction of the new hospital, the key factors driving the health system to undertake its projects were increasing digitization in healthcare, continuous improvement efforts, stringent regulatory requirements, and the need to develop and market competitive care packages. These projects faced numerous challenges in planning, due-date performance, status visibility, cost containment, and resource availability.

According to Maasstad Ziekenhuis CEO Paul Smits, the "number of concurrent projects . . . [was] cut in half due to choking the release of new projects and accelerating project completion" after implementing critical chain. By carefully managing the load on critical resources, the health system was able to avoid bad multitasking and focus "on finishing projects instead of starting them." The organization applied critical chain and included such concepts as planning each project's deliverables rather than planning each project's tasks. Constraints Management stresses that planning and measurements should be done in consideration of ultimate objectives rather than milestones on the way to the ultimate objective. By planning and measuring each project's deliverables instead of tasks, partial credit cannot be awarded for failed projects that have little benefit to the organization.

To further harness the benefits of critical chain, Maasstad Ziekenhuis set up a project board to select, plan, release, monitor, and sustain projects in monthly meetings of all supradepartmental project sponsors. With the support of senior management using the critical chain methodology, the health system's employees were able to double their monthly rate of project completion, "project lead time . . . [was] cut in half," and more than "95 percent of projects finished on time . . . [and within] scope and budget."

It is well known that software development and other IT projects are in high demand throughout the healthcare industry as treatments become more complex and medical records become electronic. After Eli Lilly & Co. applied critical chain to manage its IT group's projects, it began a pilot program in its pharmaceutical laboratories that concluded with "stupendous" results. Consequently, the Fortune 500 pharmaceutical company decided to use critical chain to manage every single product it has under development— approximately 190 projects, some that are six years long with 4,000 to 5,000 tasks. Its managers believe that "project management . . . is critical to the success of the complex, multiyear drug development process," and critical chain will give the organization a distinct competitive advantage.

Eli Lilly became convinced of the power of critical chain when its success rate in reaching project milestones on time improved to 100 percent from its 60 percent past average. John C. Lechleiter, CEO of Eli Lilly, described a pivotal point in the company's history when it entrusted its launch of a center of excellence to "streamline the development of new medicines with one common operating system, one common set of priorities, and a singular focus." Critical chain was credited not only as a pillar of the center of excellence but also with transforming Eli Lilly's relationships with clinical research organizations and other external providers.

It is difficult to deny that the process of creating lifesaving medicine is intricate and fraught with uncertainty. Yet these characteristics argue even more for the aptness of critical chain's approach because it provides a method to cope with handling the complexity, variability, and unpredictability inherent to drug-development projects. The managers of Eli Lilly have demonstrated their confidence that the company's winning formula will be found through the use of critical chain strategy and tactics.

Finance and Measures

"Throughput potential is infinite; cost savings, at some point, eats the flesh off your bone."

—CHRIS ZEPHRO, THROUGHPUT DECISION-SUPPORT EXPERT

Healthcare is expensive. This claim has become so commonplace that it seems no discussion about healthcare is complete without mentioning its cost. While the severity of the financial crisis in healthcare is reported widely in the United States, even countries with more socialized health systems are heavily burdened by high expenditures in treating patients. Whether it is a government, an insurance company, or an individual—somebody must pay, and ultimately, it is us as a society. An economist once said, "There is no such thing as a free lunch." Had he been a patient, he might also have said, "There is no such thing as free healthcare." On some level, we all pay for healthcare.

If costs are high and we all pay for healthcare, then it might follow that the primary issue facing healthcare is to reduce costs. While the impact costs have on healthcare delivery and outcomes is undeniable, concentrating primarily on costs is somewhat shortsighted. Reducing costs is not necessarily the same thing as increasing a hospital's financial well-being: Financial viability includes revenue as well as costs. As long as revenues cover costs, the relevancy of costs diminishes because a hospital's overall financial viability is ensured.

Rather than focus on costs only, perhaps healthcare systems should do something considered taboo—embrace that they are a business. And like all successful businesses, healthcare systems need to emphasize revenue beyond costs. If revenues increase, healthcare systems could reinvest the additional cash to provide better-quality care to their patients, expand coverage throughout communities, and increase profitability. After all, the potential to reduce costs is finite, limited by an organization's budget, whereas the potential to increase revenues is infinite, restricted only by however the market is defined.

There is evidence from multiple disciplines to suggest that a focus on costs paradoxically can increase costs. This point is illustrated by the following: Consider a clinic performing a simple x-ray process. Suppose that there are three steps (each with one resource) that all patients must go through in the x-ray service process. And suppose that registration takes 10 minutes, the x-ray scan takes 20 minutes, and billing/discharge takes 5 minutes, as shown in Figure 2.14.

A "cost world" mentality would be to try to improve each component of the process to reap cumulative savings. Such thinking, as is widespread today, would have little difficulty justifying a one-time expenditure to implement a new billing system that saves two minutes, reducing the final step of the process to a total of three minutes. Payback period would be calculated by dividing the cost of the improvement by the rate for two minutes of the

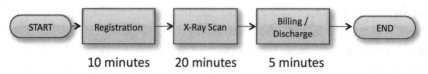

10 minutes   20 minutes   5 minutes

Figure 2.14   Process flow diagram: x-ray process example.

billing associate's time (the rate for one minute equals the billing associate's annual salary divided by the minutes he or she works in a year) multiplied by the number of patients seen by the x-ray clinic per day:

$$\text{Payback period} = \frac{\text{Cost of improvement}}{\left(\dfrac{\text{Billing associate's annual salary}}{\text{\# minutes billing associate works per year}}\right) \times \dfrac{\text{\# minutes saved by billing associate per patient}}{} \times \dfrac{\text{\# patients seen by x-ray clinic per day}}{}}$$

If the payback period, return on investment (ROI), or net present value (NPV) were favorable, the new billing system would be approved. This example seems unexceptional and rather ordinary in today's healthcare world.

However, the bottom-line impact of the new billing system is worth examining. The cost appears as an Operating Expense on the clinic's bottom line, yet no positive effect can be found elsewhere on the bottom line—no new revenue is brought in as a result of the improvement because the same number of patients were treated as before, and the billing associate's salary remains unchanged. Thus the ROI of the new billing system is negative.

If the capacity of the resources for each step of the process is analyzed using value-stream mapping—registration (6 patients per hour), x-ray scan (3 patients per hour), and billing per discharge (12 patients per hour before, 20 patients per hour after)—it becomes apparent that the x-ray scan step limits the number of patients that can be serviced overall, and therefore, this limitation determines the clinic's potential revenue, as shown in Figure 2.15. No patients can flow through the entire system faster than the x-ray scan step can process them. Assuming that there is ample demand for the clinic's services, improving the x-ray scan step of the process by increasing the number of patients who can undergo x-ray scanning per hour is the only way to grow revenue by changing the capacity of steps in this process. The x-ray scan step is the only step that, if improved, will not just benefit that local clinic but also benefit the entire process globally. Improvements

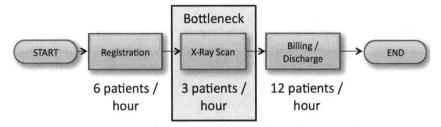

Figure 2.15   Bottleneck analysis: x-ray process example.

to this step allow more patients to be serviced by the overall system. This improvement would be reflected in the clinic's bottom-line financial viability because not only would its cost be represented as Operating Expense, but an increase in profit also would be visible as well owing to the increased number of patients using the clinic's services.

Given that a manager's attention is limited, improvement efforts should be focused on areas that have a global, system-wide impact in assisting a healthcare organization reach its goal. In the x-ray example, one way of measuring the process in relation to the goal of the clinic is the number of successful outputs, that is, patients with completed x-rays. This rate of output corresponds to the traditional definition of the Throughput of a system as developed in Constraints Management. The Constraints Management definition of Throughput will be reviewed later, but this meaning will be sufficient in this context.

As defined earlier, the factor in a process that inhibits it from reaching its goal and achieving more Throughput is called a *constraint*. In this case, since the constraint is a resource, the x-ray machine, the constraint is called a *bottleneck*. This example demonstrated that improving the billing system, a nonbottleneck, did not improve the Throughput of the overall x-ray clinic's service process. Rather, it caused only a local improvement. Goldratt also stated, "An hour saved at a nonbottleneck is a mirage." In other words, an improvement without a system impact is no improvement at all. For example, in an eight-hour workday, the x-ray clinic could service only 24 patients no matter whether the billing system is improved or not. Hence, speeding up the billing step does not affect the overall Throughput of the system.

While not ignoring that there are costs that have a global effect on processes and organizations, Constraints Management encourages a shift in emphasis from the *cost world* to the *Throughput world*. To illustrate the difference in the two paradigms of thinking, Goldratt made an analogy of organizations as chains, where each link represents a department. The cost world looks at the weight of each department. If one department reduces its costs, its link becomes lighter, and the collective weight of the chain lightens accordingly. This is how the cost world perspective thinks.

In contrast, the Throughput world looks at the strength of the chain. If one department improves its Throughput, its link strengthens. But does the entire chain strengthen? Since the strength of the chain is determined by its weakest link, it is only by improving the weakest link that the entire chain's strength can increase. Constraints Management brings a clarifying focus to improvement: Target the weakest link, the constraint, instead of targeting everything. A systems approach directed at reliability, growth, enhancement, and expansion achieved through focused thinking processes, Constraints Management–based methods strive for increased Throughput as the primary means of improvement rather than cutting costs only. Focusing on cost only will never improve the strength of the chain. Cost world thinking causes problems because it considers how to do the same with less, whereas Throughput world thinking shifts the emphasis to doing more with the same, as Kevin Watson attests.

A cost world orientation also can increase costs in encouraging policies for local efficiencies. In the x-ray clinic example, *if* there were no uncertainty and patient flow were perfectly balanced, the capacity utilization of the registration clerk would be 50 percent (the three patient per hour capacity of system divided by the six patient per hour capacity of registration clerk). If only local costs were considered and a manager wanted to improve efficiency, the manager might have the clerk process three more patients per hour to make him or her 100 percent efficient. To do so, though, would be a foolish decision because if more than three patients per hour enter the x-ray clinic, all they will do is register and wait in a queue for the x-ray scan step to occur. Even if it is unconventional to think of people as inventory, in applying management science terms to this case, adding patients increases work-in-process inventory. There is a cost associated with patient dissatisfaction as a result of long waits. Thus an increase in inventory is an increase in costs. It can be advantageous to manage strategic buffers of inventory in the real world to protect against uncertainty and variability. More about balancing flow and buffer management can be found in the supply-chain logistics section.

Even if it is not accepted that financial viability is at least part of the goal for all healthcare systems, it would be quite extreme to suggest that there is no role whatsoever for financial analysis in healthcare. One of the problems with the way fiscal analysis has been applied is that, like other businesses, many healthcare organizations use cost accounting and the same principles of allocation required for compliance with generally accepted accounting principles (GAAP) reporting standards to make financial decisions. Constraints Management promotes *Throughput accounting*, which is a special type of variable cost accounting that can be found within the managerial accounting body of knowledge. However, we prefer to call it *Throughput decision support* because it is a decision-support tool that combines the direct and variable costing aspects of managerial accounting with a focus on managing the constraint. And calling it *Throughput accounting* increases the risk of misconception that it replaces all the other financial techniques used by chief financial officers. Throughput decision-support tools are helpful for decisions on whether to add or drop services, whether to accept or reject patients covered by insurance/government reimbursement rates, where to direct marketing efforts, which projects to select, and many other areas.

Throughput decision support is not intended to replace GAAP nor the Financial Accounting Standards Board (FASB) in financial reporting. Its purpose is to provide information to supplement financial decisions. In her book, *The Measurement Nightmare*, Debra Smith illustrates the simplicity in GAAP/Throughput decision-support reconciliation, demonstrating the differences in the timing and absorption of fixed costs, as well as the valuation of inventory.

An additional advantage of Throughput decision support is that it can validate the performance of a system, whereas conventional financial measures may not detect improvements. Achieved gains even may show up as a decline in performance. For example, traditionally, an asset is defined as any good for which an expected benefit can be derived. Thus increasing inventory generally is promoted as desirable—more goods to sell in the future. Yet simply creating piles of excessive inventory to just sit on warehouse shelves, expiring and becoming obsolete, is *undesirable*. Furthermore, if management pacifies supply-chain variability with strategic buffering, along with a well-implemented replenishment strategy and, as a result, less safety stock needed to be kept on hand, the resulting reduction of inventory would appear as a decrease in assets on a balance sheet and likely would hurt the organization's perceived financial position. Therefore, a word of caution: If an organization's CEO and CFO do not fully grasp Throughput decision-support measures, performance-improvement efforts may be viewed as a failure without the right measuring system to appreciate their results.

Throughput decision support uses three global measures: Throughput (T), Investment/Inventory (I), and Operating Expense (OE). It has been noted that Constraints Management's definition of Throughput, the rate of production of goal units, is the same as the rate a for-profit business produces its contribution margin—sales revenue minus any totally variable costs (TVCs). *Totally variable costs* (TVC; a.k.a. *truly variable costs* a.k.a. *real variable costs*) are the costs to an organization that change in direct proportion to the number of units or services sold. Similar to Dr. Wadwa's definition, which was presented earlier, Motwani and colleagues define *Throughput* as "the rate at which the organization receives . . . revenues from selling medical services" or "healthcare payments in return for a patient's well-being, minus any totally variable costs directly related to these inputs."

By defining Throughput as a rate, it can be expressed for a given time period such as per month, week, day, or even minute. If the goal units are measured in money, Throughput will be an amount of money per time period. In this case, Throughput is calculated as revenues received minus totally variable costs divided by the chosen time period. A not-for-profit organization has the option to refer to *financial* Throughput, which would be defined identically to Throughput in a for-profit company. Regardless of what it is called, financial Throughput *matters*. Recall that not-for-profits are just as susceptible to a financial constraints as for-profits. Financial viability is a necessary condition to remaining open. The days of operating in the negative for years funded primarily by taxpayer subsidies are over.

Although money has been the most widely acceptable common denominator ever invented for approximating value, its applicability in healthcare to make life or death decisions can evoke passionate debate. Determination of value varies greatly among stakeholder groups—most evident are the differing perspectives between the payer and those receiving care. Even Goldratt's views evolved. Long before his recent passing, he declared that the goal of an organization is to be an *"ever flourishing* company continuously and significantly increasing value to stakeholders— employees, clients, and shareholders.

In summary, a not-for-profit should search out and correct the causes of the undesirable effects (UDEs) affecting Throughput while keeping the costs of Investment and Operating Expense down. But the primary emphasis always should be on the former, not the latter. Constraints Management promotes maximization of the Throughput (T) first, then reduction of Investment/Inventory (I), and finally reduction of Operating Expenses (OE). This prioritization is a major paradigm shift, as seen in the relative emphasis of management philosophies in Figure 2.16 on page 88.

In the book, *The Haystack Syndrome*, Goldratt defines *Investment* or *Inventory* (I) as all the money the system invests in purchasing things the system intends to sell. This meaning expands on traditional categories of inventory (i.e., raw materials, work in process, and finished goods) to also include capital assets, facilities, equipment, and receivables. *Operating Expense* (OE) is defined as all the money the organization spends in generating goal units/Throughput—the money flowing out of the system. OE is all the money spent turning I into T. Normally, most categories of overhead are considered to be fixed over a short time horizon and are designated as Operating Expense. OE includes all the money an organization would pay, even if production or service were to stop for a while, such as salaries, rent, insurance, depreciation, energy, food services, security, maintenance/repair, and janitorial services.

Indirect Measures

$$\text{Net profit} = T - OE$$

$$\text{ROI} = \frac{T - OE}{I}$$

$$\text{Productivity} = \frac{T}{OE}$$

$$\text{Investment turns} = \frac{T}{I}$$

$$\text{Cash flow} = T - OE - \Delta I$$

where T, I, and OE are the total Throughput, Investment (or Inventory) and Operating Expense of the system.

Another strength of Throughput decision support is that when it comes time to making decisions, it makes it easy to separate the totally variable

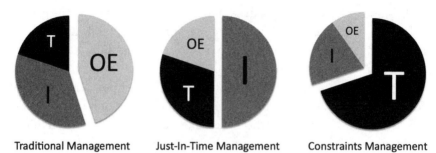

Traditional Management   Just-In-Time Management   Constraints Management

Figure 2.16   The relative emphasis of management philosophies.

costs from fixed costs rather than trying to allocate fixed cost as variable costs based on some arbitrary driver, as is typical under full absorption cost accounting and ABC accounting. Once management makes the decision to maintain adequate staffing to keep the day-to-day business of a hospital operating, regardless of the number of patients treated, general fixed costs are sunk costs and therefore become irrelevant during decision making and consequently should not be absorbed into the cost of services. Using direct labor as a driver for overhead allocation may have made sense in the past, but Ronen and colleagues point out that two things have changed. First, labor has become more of a fixed cost than a variable cost because piece-rate work has become less ubiquitous. Second, overhead has grown from 5 to 10 percent of the cost of production in the 1920s to 20 to 80 percent of the cost of production today.

Let us go back to our example and assume that there is a new constraint back at the x-ray clinic. This time, the constraint is a market constraint, and it reveals itself because the clinic treats only one patient per hour on average, reducing the system's capacity to one-third its potential (recall that the bottleneck's capacity is three patients per hour). The clinic receives $80 for providing x-ray services to each patient covered by private insurance. Salaries for the employees, rent for the clinic, utilities, janitorial services, x-ray machine maintenance, and depreciation are allocated at an overhead rate of $50 per patient according to cost accounting absorption principles. The $20 that is allocated for radiographic film and other developing materials, envelopes, and paper gowns is classified as a totally variable cost per patient because this expense is incurred incrementally as patient volume increases.

The clinic calculates its net revenues as $10 per patient: $80 of private insurance reimbursement minus $70 of absorbed cost ($50 of overhead plus

$20 of totally variable costs for each patient). When faced with the choice of accepting patients covered by public health insurance at a reimbursement rate of $55, the clinic calculates a prospective loss of $15 per patient: $55 of government insurance reimbursement minus $70 of absorbed (or fully burdened) cost, as shown in Table 2.4. Therefore, the clinic's management will conclude that the clinic loses money by treating patients with public health insurance, such as Medicaid, and ultimately will decide to decline those patients if they have that option.

Table 2.4   Accept a Loss?

	Private Insurance	Public Health Insurance
Revenue	$80	$55
Totally variable costs	–$20	–$20
Overhead	–$50	–$50
	$10 gain	$15 loss

From a financial perspective, the decision not to accept patients with public health insurance would be reasonable, but the decision should take the market constraint the clinic faces into consideration. If the clinic could have filled its capacity treating three patients each hour with private insurance, it would have made more money than if it had treated any patients with public health insurance. However, analysis of this example using Throughput decision support, or even managerial accounting fundamentals, reveals that the clinic should have accepted patients insured by the government. Here is the explanation: Given that the clinic had already made the commitment to keep its doors open and pay its rent, salaries, utilities, and so on, those costs were sunk costs and therefore should not have played into the decision whether to accept patients with public health insurance.

Since the clinic was treating only one patient per hour owing to low demand, paid resources were *unnecessarily* idle because the clinic chose *not* to accept patients with public health insurance. Hence, as long as the public health insurance reimbursement covered the totally variable costs of treating each patient while fewer than three privately insured patients per hour demanded the clinic's services, the clinic should have accepted patients with public health insurance. Covering totally variable costs can be defined as whatever margin makes business sense to the healthcare organization.

Any price received over the totally variable cost would contribute toward either paying fixed expense or increased profits and thus should be accepted. A hospital's financial viability should not be put at risk if it treats more patients: The more patients it treats, the more financially viable the hospital should be. After all, if the hospital no longer exists in the future, it cannot heal *anybody*.

As long as any insurance reimbursement covered the totally variable costs of treating each patient plus some acceptable margin, and less than three privately insured patients per hour demanded its services, from a purely financial perspective, the clinic should have accepted patients with such insurance. Throughput decision support can help financial managers to follow the real money. In the terminology of Constraints Management, decisions that increase Throughput are *good* for the organization. Efforts to reduce Inventory/Investment and Operating Expenses are also encouraged, but not at the expense of Throughput. In the preceding example, $55 revenue per patient with public insurance minus $20 totally variable costs per patient yielded a Throughput of $35 per patient, whereas the clinic's bottom-line Investment and Operating Expense did not change, as shown in Table 2.5.

Table 2.5 Bottom-Line Impact

	Public Health Insurance
Revenue	$55
Totally Variable Costs	–$20
Throughput	$35
Investment	(No change)
Operating Expense	(No change)
	$35 gain

Distributing fixed costs across services distorts the true cost of services and hence interferes with decision making. Reviews of traditional cost measurements have exposed the direct link between traditional measures and missed due dates, excessive expediting, and long lead times. It has been said, "Tell me how you measure me and I will tell you how I will behave." If an organization's measurement system does not reinforce and incentivize achievement of the goal, it undermines its own interests.

A global perspective can challenge traditionally local views. This perspective reveals that it is not always appropriate to classify inventory as an asset in decision making. When inventory is mismatched with what is needed, whether stocked out, overstocked, or perishable, inventory can act as a liability. The cost of inventory should be treated as what it really is—the cost in buffering against uncertainty. The real power of a system approach is harnessed when it is combined with a *Throughput world* framework. Such a union can make evident that across-the-board cost cuts are undesirable not just because they hurt the sprint/protective capacity of nonbottleneck resources in recovering from Murphy (special-cause variation) and keep cycle times down but also because they cut the constrained resource, which effectively restricts the output of the system.

Conclusion

Like the Lean archetype's seven deadly wastes, understanding the constraints of a system is akin to wearing glasses, allowing focus on what is responsible for the worst kind of waste—the wasted opportunity to reach the goal. Just as Lean urges that waste be attacked anywhere it is found, Constraints Management similarly compels that constraints be managed anywhere they are found. Artificial constraints should be broken anywhere they are encountered. System constraints can never be eliminated—only relocated. And as Chris Zephro has remarked, "*Real constraints* are not good or bad; they just are, so either you manage them or *they manage you.*"

Managers always should aspire to move the constraint of any system to a strategically desirable place. Assuming that they are strategically relevant, constraints such as resources, the market, and policies that stand in the way of goal attainment should be managed carefully. Constraints Management warns to never be complacent and to always dynamically adjust to an ever-changing environment, avoiding inertia.

The way Constraints Management works is that it allows practitioners to simplify complexity by revealing the interdependencies of systems. Strategic and tactical leverage points are revealed so that managers know where to concentrate their local efforts to achieve the greatest global improvement. Constraints Management encompasses a multidisciplinary toolset that facilitates performance improvement in a number of applications. Its applications can be used in strategic development, service and production logistics, supply chains, project management, finance, measures, and others.

▲ Buffer management provides a mechanism to respond dynamically and adapt to variation in demand and supply to maximize Throughput for an organization.

▲ Logistics solutions facilitate getting the most out of the bottlenecks, whether they exist in supply chains or internal operations.

▲ Critical chain eliminates multitasking and resource contention and fosters trust and good communications to complete projects dramatically faster and within budget.

▲ Throughput decision support sheds light on what actually affects the bottom line and what is simply a local improvement without any global benefit to an organization and a measurement system that supports that aim.

As powerful as its preexisting applications are, Constraints Management also allows unique solutions tailored to the specific situations that organizations experience. Constraints Management demonstrates how to harness our intuition and transform our thinking processes to develop commonsense, breakthrough, win-win solutions where the root causes of issues are eliminated. Its fundamental philosophy is humanistic and persistently strives for growth and Throughput rather than cutting costs as the means of improvement.

Constraints Management provides a mechanism to highlight leverage points, or weakest links, where efforts should be concentrated so that focused performance improvement can be attained. Constraints Management combines effectively with other tools. Lean and Six Sigma tools can be used to identify and get the most out of the constraints. Constraints Management tools also can be used within Six Sigma's DMAIC roadmap as well as in value-stream analyses and rapid improvement workshops. An organization cannot truly be Lean without being aware of and managing its constraints. And Constraints Management, Six Sigma, and Lean need each other, and they are further boosted with innovation tools such as TRIZ.

Although Constraints Management is in its infancy in healthcare, its potential is immense, as has been demonstrated in its early applications and confirmed experientially in other industries. While it has been known that the contributions of Constraints Management are especially adept in logistics and resource planning, its promise as a strategic tool for healthcare organizations has been, as of yet, largely unrealized. Since, by definition, there is at least one constraint in every organization, and because it is impossible to break every constraint, constraints must be managed. Constraints Management requires understanding of the big-picture interactions and fluctuations—systems thinking, in short. There has never been a more opportune time to use Constraints Management to better manage healthcare systems.

CHAPTER 3

An Integrated Approach to Deploying Performance Improvement

As it relates to performance improvement, the term *deployment* has come to mean different things to different people. Regardless of how it is defined, it is widely accepted that, as with any organizational change effort, a plan is essential. To some of those who do develop a deployment plan, it is little more than a training schedule; to others, it may include a list of processes that require improvement. To facilitate a successful deployment, it must be both of these and much more. The deployment plan should provide a roadmap to a successful and sustainable performance-improvement program. It should clearly address the strategy for how performance improvement will be used to facilitate the attainment of organizational goals today and in the future. It is not an easy task, but the rewards are well worth the effort.

Who Leads the Performance-Improvement Deployment?

While the deployment plan sets the path for the journey, someone must lead the way. Most successful deployments appoint a *deployment champion*. The deployment champion should be an executive-level leader (e.g., chief quality officer, vice president for performance improvement, etc.). At a minimum, deployment champions should have a working knowledge of performance-improvement tools and techniques. If possible, they should attend practitioner training. While it is optimal for them to complete projects as is normally required for practitioner courses, this may be waived—allowing the champion to attend much in the same manner a student may audit a college course. While not the favored approach, this may be preferred over a void in performance-improvement knowledge.

The primary duty of deployment champions is to execute the deployment strategy. This is accomplished through the *executive leadership team* (ELT). Many healthcare organizations have multiple entities that oversee, report, or execute improvement efforts across the enterprise—or even within departments. While this ubiquity does help to ensure a degree of focus on quality issues, it is somewhat counter to a systems approach to quality throughout the organization. For the Committee on Quality of Health Care in America, the Institute of Medicine (IOM) stated that "whatever the organizational arrangement, it should promote innovation and quality improvement." Top-level management ought to ask, "Does the current decentralized structure promote innovation and sharing?" Additionally, the IOM found that a healthcare organization's structure must be able to support both formal and informal ways of learning to share information. Otherwise, improvements will be suboptimized, with improvements limited to just one division or team instead of reaped throughout the organization, as Samantha Chao attests in her report, "The State of Quality Improvement and Implementation Research."

In many cases, relegating the responsibility of quality outside the highest echelon of management serves to absolve executive leadership from direct involvement in improving quality within their organization. While the focus of these entities is usually on quality-of-care issues, the organization's raison d'être, it fails to address opportunities in the areas of capacity, Throughput, and cost containment. These multiple quality entities are representative of the organizational silos that are widespread in healthcare.

Performance-Improvement Program Management Office

In performance improvement, initiatives undertaken to mitigate performance gaps are generally called *projects*. This nomenclature can be confusing when reviewing literature regarding *project* or *program* management. In some cases, they are treated synonymously. In this book, the term *project* is used when discussing individual improvement undertakings, and *program* is used when addressing the overall performance-improvement deployment.

Establishing a program office is an immediate responsibility of the executive leadership team. It is necessary to provide oversight and program management. At a minimum, this office should be responsible for the administrative tasks in support of the performance-improvement deployment. Ideally, senior practitioners should be centralized and be assigned to the program management office to work on performance improvement full time. Their role should be to provide technical oversight and deployment advice and to lead improvement efforts that affect the strategic goals of the organization. To quantify the impact of these efforts, as well as more localized efforts within work units, the deployment champion, as the head of the program office, should coordinate with the finance department to develop and implement a benefit estimation and validation process—when the *JumpStart* process is applied, this task is accomplished by the deployment team. JumpStart is a rapid planning process developed to accomplish a large amount of performance-improvement planning in a very short time with the executive leadership team. The use of centralized management offices is a quickly growing concept in businesses worldwide.

Depending on the maturity level of the healthcare organization, the program office may be responsible for the delivery of all training related to performance improvement. In the earlier stages of the performance-improvement deployment, the program office provides for the availability of external resources contracted to deliver the training. Regardless of its maturity level, an organization may decide that outsourcing the delivery of training remains a viable option.

In addition to being the principal of the program office, the deployment champion is also responsible for maintaining the project portfolio, which lists improvement opportunities throughout the organization, as well as management of project selection and prioritization processes. While project identification and prioritization are executive leadership functions, the deployment champion must be active in advising and coaching executives. The deployment champion continuously monitors progress toward milestones and performance relative to indicators, reporting exceptions to executive leadership.

Prioritization

Addressed in more detail in Chapter 5, project prioritization is a critical component of any performance-improvement deployment. One key contribution of Constraints Management to the integrated approach is the use of thinking processes tools to identify and prioritize improvement opportunities with the potential for a system-level impact. It is important to determine whether an improvement opportunity affects the system constraint or at least one of the core drivers of a top-level undesirable effect. The current reality tree (CRT) and its simplified version, the focused current reality tree (fCRT), reveal the leverage points and opportunities that yield the greatest potential for a healthcare organization to progress toward attainment of its goal. CRTs can bring the core drivers to the surface and provide the framework to discover the actions that best mitigate them.

In the approach, the linkage between core drivers and improvement opportunities cannot be overstated. In addition, agreement with strategic imperatives, as well as performance gaps related to regulatory requirements, voluntary accreditations, and annual reviews of key performance indicators, are considered. Cost, quality, and time assessments of core processes are conducted. Although financial impact is critical, estimates of expected benefits also should be provided in other areas, such as patient safety and clinical outcomes, with weights that the executive team deems as important components of project selection and prioritization.

Long-term success depends on the routine direct involvement of executive leadership in performance improvement. The execution of the strategy and guidance provided by the executive leadership team should be concentrated in a program management office. The deployment champion advises the executive leadership team on how to integrate and align the performance-improvement program with organizational strategy.

Initiating a performance-improvement deployment can be a time-consuming process. Forming the program management office is a critical first step. The next step is to form a deployment team and initiate assessment and planning as rapidly as possible.

Deployment Team

The deployment team is formed during the early phase of the deployment. Its members include management representatives from

▲ Program management office
▲ Executive leadership team
▲ Patient care

▲ Public affairs/community relations
▲ Human resources/organizational development
▲ Finance

The anticipated life cycle of the team as a distinct entity typically is no longer than through the initial stages of the deployment. Team members may have individual tasks stemming from the deployment plan or may be contacted to provide input on matters within their areas of expertise. Over time, these areas of responsibility will be absorbed by the deployment champion and program management office.

What Does a Mature Hospital Performance-Improvement Deployment Look Like?

There are many facets to a mature, successful performance-improvement deployment in a hospital. Governance, staffing, finance, and visibility are four crucial features of a performance-improvement deployment.

Governance

Governance of the performance-improvement program is a shared responsibility. At the strategic level, executive leadership identifies strategic goals and allocates resources to mitigate gaps. Executive leadership actively participates in the prioritization of projects focused on strategic goals or those that cross the enterprise. Next, the tactical level is the responsibility of the healthcare organization's quality leader (e.g., vice president for quality improvement). The quality leader sets the policies and advises other executives on the progress of the performance-improvement program. Policies are to be established covering project identification, prioritization, monitoring, execution, and reporting.

At the operational level, centrally assigned practitioners aligned organizationally under the quality leader should be expected to complete between four and eight high-impact/high-visibility projects per year. These projects should be focused on areas having the potential for a high return on investment and/or a direct impact on strategic objectives. Additionally, the centralized core of practitioners provides mentoring and project oversight to decentralized practitioners. These decentralized practitioners continue to work in their normal jobs and assist their managers in identification and execution of performance-improvement events within their departments or divisions.

A single tracking system should be used to capture information related to all performance-improvement projects completed within the organization regardless of the level of sponsorship or the toolset applied. All performance-improvement projects are to be formally chartered, including a clearly articulated business case along with a validation of the operational improvements, revenue increases, and cost savings achieved after the improved process is implemented. Before long, active participation in the performance-improvement program should be regarded as an expectation for career progression within the organization.

Staffing

At least one full-time practitioner is dedicated to the execution of high-impact, cross-departmental projects. Other decentralized, *at-large practitioners* are available for departmental projects. These at-large practitioners are expected to complete one to two projects per year, generally within their department or work unit. An ongoing program of performance-improvement training is established beginning with the executive team and progressing downward in the organization. All leaders should be trained to sponsor improvement projects. At maturity, frontline supervisors sponsor improvement efforts led by practitioners to improve processes under their operational purview. Every person who attends practitioner training and remains assigned within his or her respective work unit should lead at least two improvement events per year, such as a process value-stream analysis, rapid improvement workshop, or 5S events, which are explained in Chapter 5. An ongoing training program should result in no fewer than one trained practitioner in every department/work unit of the hospital.

Finance

The finance department, under the direction of the chief financial officer (CFO), must establish procedures for its active participation in establishing the business case for projects, as well as estimation and validation of cost savings and revenues to be achieved on completion of performance-improvement projects. Chapter 7 describes the process for estimation and validation of financial benefits of performance-improvement projects and events. Interdepartmental reports are maintained to document the cumulative return on investment (ROI) of the organization's performance-improvement program. The results demonstrate that performance improvement is not a cost center—but rather a profit center—for the organization.

Visibility

All employees should be introduced to the performance-improvement program during their orientation as new employees to the healthcare organization. Responsibility is rotated through the team so that each senior leader presents. Performance-improvement successes must be publicized and celebrated at every opportunity. In addition to regular publication in organizational newsletters or announcement via some other means, each project team prepares a storyboard and displays it in the benefitting work center. In the United States, it is common to see these storyboards maintained and used for a performance-improvement storyboard gallery each year during national quality month and/or presented at regional and national meetings such as those of the Institute for Healthcare Improvement (IHI) and National Association for Healthcare Quality (NAHQ). This should be encouraged as a means of recognizing practitioners and promoting benchmarking and sharing of best practices. One or two performance-improvement projects at a minimum are presented each month at the executive team meeting. These projects are introduced by the respective sponsor and presented by the lead practitioner. The CFO regularly presents the ROI statistics on the overall performance-improvement program. On a quarterly basis, a high-visibility project is presented to the board of directors.

Nondelegable Responsibilities of Leadership

"The four hardest jobs in America (not necessarily in order) are: President of the United States, a university president, a hospital CEO, and a pastor."
—PETER DRUCKER, WRITER, PROFESSOR, AND MANAGEMENT GURU

The role of executive leadership in any deployment or organizational change effort is nondelegable. It cannot be reassigned to others with any reasonable assurance of success. While it is tempting to expansively task individuals with focusing their efforts on changing the way the organization operates, it won't last more than a few months—six months at the maximum. Changing the way an organization thinks, handles information, collects data, and manages its operational processes is a daunting task even in less turbulent times. Today's healthcare environment isn't exactly smooth sailing.

There is much about tomorrow, next week, and next month that is unknown. Healthcare reform, changes in payer reimbursement, increased requirements for greater accountability and performance at lower cost, and congressional pressure for greater access to care—all are a significant part of the unknown and contribute to the enormous amount of environmental uncertainty in the marketplace.

Only members of the executive team have the positional authority and visibility necessary to drive change despite this instability. Thus it is imperative that executive leaders take the helm themselves and safely guide their organization. What distinguishes executive leaders from others is what they can do from their position in the organization. Executive leaders can

▲ Understand what works well in their organization

▲ Be aware of areas that demand their further attention

▲ Have sufficient courage and strength to undertake the most appropriate risks needed to enact the required changes

▲ Know what resources are available to create the change

▲ Provide rewards and recognition to appropriately incentivize and acknowledge their employees

▲ Have the power to create the impulse to change and drive it through the organization

Instituting any new methodology, skill, or expertise, such as those required for performance improvement, entails understanding what currently works well in the organization and what does not. Unless someone can see where the successes and failures exist, any form of improvement will be short-lived. Perhaps previous efforts to introduce new tools and methodologies have met with limited success and resulted in temporary, quick fixes. Quite possibly the staff has become so used to "flavor of the month" programs that it will ignore any new methodology regardless of how well it is presented. In any case, deciphering what is happening within the organization and where improvements are needed is always vested in executive leadership. It requires simultaneous big-picture thinking and attention to specific details. This perspective is difficult to achieve without having the wide array of experiences achieved by those at the top of the pyramid. There is no substitute for the time-tested, highly experienced, and battle-hardened executive who can see the forest *and* the trees simultaneously.

In addition to understanding what works well and having the wealth of experiences to execute, there is a need for the ability to take risks when and where appropriate. Implementing a new way of viewing the organization's people, processes, and resources and making change happen involves significant risk-taking. Many hospital executives have attempted to implement performance-improvement initiatives only to have them fail—or they had some initial successes and then lost steam, realizing fewer and fewer results as time went on. Taking risks is not for the faint of heart. It requires knowledge, understanding, tact, confidence, and perseverance— all of which are the qualities necessary for a leader to be successful. Each is required to implement performance improvement successfully. The literature cited throughout this book well illustrates the successes achieved by numerous hospitals, universities, and medical centers. Yet they were not achieved without the executive leadership taking the time to assess the risks and committing the time, money, and people necessary to be successful.

Executive leaders achieve much of their success by using the right resources, at the right time, with the right amount of motivation, and when milestones are achieved, providing the appropriate recognition and rewards. Implementing, growing, and sustaining a performance-improvement program requires this careful mix of the resources, motivation, and recognition. Get the mixture wrong, and the program dies quickly from lack of sustainment or micromanagement. Overdoing the mixture is just as harmful as doing too little. Sustainment requires executive leadership to be on top of their performance-improvement activities, continuously monitoring results and providing the right resources to make any needed midcourse corrections without succumbing to micromanagement.

Burning Platform

Piper Alpha was a North Sea oil production platform operated by Occidental Petroleum that caught fire and was destroyed on July 6, 1988, killing 167 men, with only 59 survivors. At the time, one of the workers was trapped by the fire on the edge of the platform. Rather than certain death in the fire, he chose probable death by jumping 100 feet into the freezing sea. He survived. This tragedy on a *burning platform* has evolved into the business lexicon, meaning that immediate and radical change is necessary owing to dire circumstances. Another name for this is a *personal inflection point*. Sometimes it is a choice; sometimes an inflection point is cast on us.

If there is one element that belongs solely to executive leadership, it is the ability to articulate and monitor the burning platform. Hospitals often find themselves in a status quo frame of mind: *Things are going well enough.* Revenue is enough to get by and make payroll. The patients appear reasonably satisfied with their level of care. The hospital successfully passes its inspections with only a few minor discrepancies. In other words, the hospital is not in a crisis mode. Unfortunately, this is all too often the setting when attempting to institute change. The need or requirement for change meets with strong resistance. The attitude of the staff is, "Why change?"

Yet today's chaotic environment requires a significant change in the way successful hospitals are to operate in the weeks, months, and years to come. Making this change, implementing new or expanded performance-improvement initiatives necessitates creating sufficient pressure or leverage that employees see that change is necessary. It is the burning platform that can quickly motivate employees out of their status quo orientation and provide the incentives to try something new. Only the executive leadership has the power, ability, and experience to create the burning platform—that *sense of urgency* necessary to stimulate dramatic organizational change. If anyone subordinate to them attempts to do it, it will quickly die out. They don't have what the executive leadership has—the power and tools to make it happen.

It is worth noting that executive leaders have only so much time to accomplish myriad of tasks, attend an endless array of meetings, and at the same time, focus on the future direction of the organization. Some tasks and occasional meetings can be delegated to others. This only makes sense. What cannot be delegated, however, is the role of leading, guiding, and sustaining performance-improvement programs. The risks are too high to be left to others in the organization. Resources, recognitions, and rewards—all are needed in due course with the correct application. The staff knows and expects this. It is the nondelegable role of executive leadership to do it right the first time and to sustain their efforts over the long term.

Transactional versus Transformational Leadership

Another way to describe the type of leadership that facilitates a successful performance-improvement deployment is *transformational leadership*. This concept, as contrasted with *transactional leadership*, was developed by Bernard Bass in 1985. A *transactional* leader is one who is responsive to immediate self-interests if they can be met by *getting the work done*. Conversely, a transformational leader raises the level of team awareness with the goal of getting the team to go beyond self-interest for the sake of the larger goal, as John B. Miner conveyed in his book, *Organizational Behavior*.

This style of leadership was thrust on the healthcare industry in 2002 when the National Health System (NHS) of Great Britain described the type of leadership required to usher in the NHS vision for the new century. In the book, *Effective Healthcare Leadership*, edited by Jasper and Jumaa, the NHS chief executive attested that leadership that set a vision and worked through people to attain it was necessary, in addition to the following skills and qualities:

▲ Broad scanning
▲ Intellectual flexibility
▲ Seizing the future
▲ Effective and strategic influencing

The leadership of the NHS saw these leadership traits as necessary to usher in major changes. They are exactly the same as those required to facilitate success at the helm of a performance-improvement deployment. These leaders need to look beyond reacting to sentinel events and forced budget reductions. They need to support the type of proactive pursuit of improvement opportunities that will preclude the occurrence of these events.

Leadership Coaching

Mentoring other, less skilled practitioners is inherent in the role of all performance-improvement practitioners. This responsibility is a fundamental competency of master practitioners. The master practitioner is a conduit for knowledge transfer. This role as an advisor or coach transcends practitioner-to-practitioner interaction (mentoring for skill development will be discussed later in the development section of Chapter 5). A coach fosters the integration of generally existing skills into a new context. Coaching includes helping leaders adapt their skills to leading in a performance-improvement-focused environment and to understanding tools and techniques, change management, and communication approaches.

Managing Upward

One crucial skill in providing leadership coaching is the ability to manage upward. To many, this is a strange concept. Most believe that management occurs downward only. In an article she wrote for the *British Journal of Hospital Medicine*, Dr. Rachel Hooke described five key points on managing upward:

▲ Be clear and assertive.
▲ Don't assume that they know the intricacies of the topic.
▲ They may be having a bad day.
▲ Know what makes them tick.
▲ Use influencing skills.

Another article from the *Financial Times* addresses some traits in leaders to facilitate a good working relationship. In it, Adrian Furnham defined a crucial overarching trait in managing upward, *fluid intelligence*—being quick on the uptake regarding new or unfamiliar information. Those lacking this fluid intelligence require more sensitive handling. Other traits that affect how one manages upward include

▲ Level of negative affectivity—how well they deal with stress
▲ Extroversion versus introversion
▲ Level of conscientiousness
▲ Agreeableness
▲ Level of curiosity and creativity

While much of the literature focuses on how to manage upward, some of the responsibility for the success of leadership coaching efforts must be placed on the leader. A commonly cited reason for less than open and honest upward communication is fear of retribution or negative career impact by the coach. In *Personnel Journal*, Gary Gemmill wrote that the leader can allay these fears by rewarding open communications and by being more open about the areas in which he or she requires assistance or guidance.

Frequently, the master practitioner needs to mentor or manage upward during the initial stages of a performance-improvement deployment. Physician involvement is critical, especially when critical inaugural projects and events are clinical in nature. It is not uncommon for the chief medical officer to "push back" when he or she realizes that a physician is expected to participate as a fully involved member of the team, not just as an ad hoc advisor. In this case, it is essential to manage expectations carefully and to reinforce that physician participation is not optional but necessary if the project is to have any chance of success. The success of the deployment can hinge on the practitioner's skill and confidence in handling this situation. Physicians who participate in events as fully engaged members of an interdisciplinary performance-improvement team can become powerful proponents for the deployment, as shown in Figure 3.1. Teams that struggle to improve processes without physician involvement often find their efforts undone after the fact. This quite effectively crushes their enthusiasm, eliminates any sense of empowerment, and poses a grave risk to the deployment. This must be made clear to executive leadership consistently and assertively from the beginning.

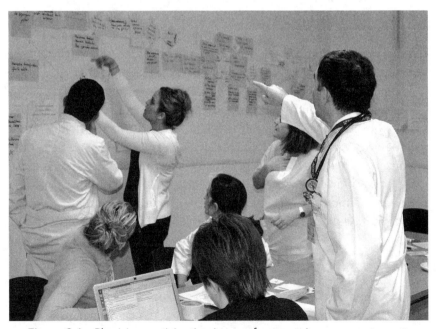

Figure 3.1 Physician participation in a performance-improvement event.

If physician participation in performance-improvement activities is to be successful, it should be focused and targeted. It is best to use physician input not only as a customer of a process but also as a driver of the process. This may require the actual presence of physicians at a performance-improvement team meeting or offline input gathered by a team member prior to the meeting. Physicians' time should be used judiciously. As one performance-improvement team found, "We just had to catch them when we could. We were determined to make the best use of the physicians' time, even if it was for a very short period of time."

Pulling physicians away from their work is not easy. However, it can be done skillfully given the correct incentives. Participation by physicians in performance improvement can be incentivized by offsetting any time dedicated with a pardon from other medical duties. This can be especially effective in very large medical centers, in which the physicians are on multiple committees. Giving them a pardon enables the performance-improvement teams to gain what is in very short supply—the physician's true perspectives on the process. Some physicians can be cross-utilized as valuable resources for a number of different clinical performance-improvement teams. For example, physicians working with utilization review and management information systems (MIS) can aggregate valuable data to support various stages of multiple improvement events. Physicians have a unique ability to quickly obtain and assess data. They can spot errors in data collection faster with their unique perspective and can skillfully help the teams gather the correct data the first time, every time.

Regardless of physician involvement, executives must be coached to understand the balance between easy solutions and solutions that are sustainable. Approaches also must balance the technical discipline of the methodology with the level of acceptance that can be anticipated across the organization. It must be aligned with the organizational culture and the underlying rationale that caused the organization to decide to undertake a performance-improvement deployment. The overall approach must be robust enough to meet the needs of the organization initially and over the long term.

What Is a Robust Deployment Approach?

A robust approach for deploying performance improvement is applicable to any organization regardless of its current degree of deployment progress or success. Three ways to categorize this progress are

CASE STUDY

Leadership Coaching

Shortly after becoming the chief executive at a major healthcare system, the CEO began receiving regular briefings on performance-improvement activities at her various hospitals and clinics. While most projects were proceeding according to plan, and goals were being met, the executive would ask deep, probing questions of the practitioners and then—in many cases—change the scope of the project midstream. While well within her jurisdiction as CEO, these adjustments were resulting in a great deal of angst on the part of the practitioners and ultimately were having an adverse affect on the progress of the performance-improvement efforts. Practitioners became reluctant to move quickly between briefs because there was a good chance that they would be redirected.

After seeing the impact that the CEO's input and involvement were having on the performance-improvement deployment, the deployment champion had a discussion with the CEO and explained that while her involvement was laudable, changing scope multiple times throughout project life cycles was having an adverse affect on overall program efficacy. After some discussion on the balance between executive prerogative and the need for project stability, the CEO decided that the best course of action was to increase her involvement in the initial chartering of enterprise-level projects. Thus her input would be heard during project planning. Lower-level projects would be briefed to her on completion.

▲ Greenfield
▲ Revitalization
▲ New heights

Every organization must decide what its purpose or goal is in deploying performance improvement. For some, it is the absence of a structured approach to performance improvement altogether. Others have an approach in place and desire to either revitalize it or take it to the next level. The most obvious level of maturity is the organization with virtually no structured approach in place. In such organizations, this is referred to as a *greenfield deployment*, and these organizations may have been realizing some degree of improvement, but it was not due to any organized or focused level of effort.

CASE STUDY

Hospital System-Level Greenfield

A not-for-profit hospital system decided to implement an integrated approach to performance improvement across their system. The existing performance-improvement program was decentralized and reactive. It consisted largely of collecting data and reporting core measures and reacting to isolated incidents. Any proactive actions were taken as a result of annual strategic planning and focused on loosely defined "initiatives." Reactions to isolated incidents were handled largely through application of the find-organize-clarify-understand-select (FOCUS)–plan-do-check-act (PDCA) strategy (the nine-step process-improvement methodology based on the work of W. Edwards Deming discussed in Chapter 1) and realized marginal success. No data were available to demonstrate long-term efficacy of FOCUS-PDCA improvement efforts. Improvements were not fully implemented or were not sustained. There was no analysis of any direct impact on patient care, and financial results were not estimated or validated. Efforts in support of annual strategic planning were broadly scoped and managed more from a local perspective than from across the entire value stream.

After a two-week JumpStart event in which a comprehensive deployment plan was developed, the organization immediately initiated a series of performance-improvement projects scoped to manageable process levels. The JumpStart was run initially by contract practitioners and quickly transitioned to trained, organic resources.

Now, more than one year into the performance-improvement deployment, the system has two full-time practitioners who lead complex projects as directed by the executive leadership team, as well as provide oversight of more than 40 practitioners trained to execute performance-improvement events at the department level.

CASE STUDY

Department-Level Greenfield Deployment

A large urban medical center had been using a standard performance-improvement methodology for several years with mixed results. While it passed Joint Commission accreditation visits successfully, the staff intuitively knew that it could do better. Moreover, there were reports that money was leaking from the system, and tracking down the specific sources of the leak was proving to be increasingly difficult. Having heard and read recent reports regarding other hospitals' successes with more rigorous approaches to performance improvement, an integrated approach was especially apt.

The first step was to conduct a *system-level value-stream analysis* (SystemVSA or SVSA) to identify the core processes and performance gaps (described later in this chapter and further in Chapter 4). The SVSA created a high-level view of the process. From this perspective, it was clear that the department suffered from problems in multiple areas, including interventional radiology. Deciding which problem to tackle was no easy decision, especially given the critical importance of interventional radiology services throughout the entire medical center and satellite hospitals. In discussions with executives, it became evident that rather than making money, it was losing cash rapidly. The interventional radiology department had recently expanded its services to include more studies and treatments with the intention of expanding services and thereby gaining greater market share, specifically in the treatment of advanced cancers.

Based on the results of the planning sessions, a process-level value-stream analysis (ProcessVSA or PVSA; introduced in Chapter 1 and detailed further in Chapter 6) for the interventional radiology diagnosis and treatment process was sponsored by the chief operating officer to understand the dynamics of the process and analyze whether each step added value to the patient, as shown in Figure 3.2. The performance-improvement team included a surgeon, an interventional radiologist, administrative clerical staff, nursing personnel, and staff from chemotherapy and nuclear medicine. An analysis of the individual

CASE STUDY

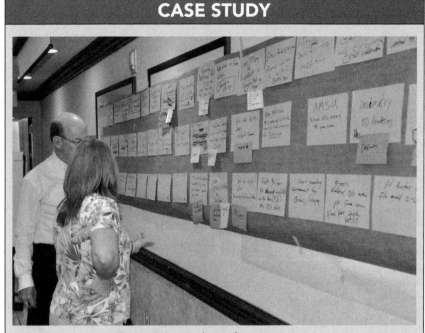

Figure 3.2 Analysis of process steps.

process steps demonstrated that many were non-value-added, and rather than helping to improve the treatment flow of the patients, the steps were creating longer and longer cycle times. Patients were increasingly frustrated with the long wait times for diagnosis and treatments. The physicians were frustrated with endless delays in having their patients registered into the hospital databases, insurance verifications, and staff preparation of their patients for the procedures.

The potential impact of the ProcessVSA became readily evident. Of the two-week total time for treatment of cancer patients, only 10 percent of the time was devoted to diagnosis, treatment, and nursing recovery. Most of the time was expended on administrative and clerical tasks. Additionally, critical steps in the coding, tracking, and billing for each patient's treatment had been overlooked or were poorly implemented. Reimbursement for several patients was simply lost. The ProcessVSA resulted in a 40 percent reduction in the non-value-added steps and in

CASE STUDY

a far more efficient treatment of patients. The ProcessVSA also revealed the bottleneck of the process—ambulatory services. A focused rapid-improvement session enabled the team to increase the capacity of the bottleneck by about 50 percent without any new investment. An improvement-opportunity portfolio was developed within the radiology department listing other opportunities, such as improving the coding and billing processes to increase reimbursement rates.

Some organizations have initiated actions to institutionalize their performance-improvement program but seem unable to gain any real traction. These *false starts* tend to create disenchantment with a focused performance-improvement program. Both organizational leadership and staff begin to believe that they were better off with whatever method or approach they were using prior to the current deployment. This is common in healthcare organizations, where many versions of quality improvement are either currently in place or have been in place over the years. Not only are several approaches being used, but they also tend to be disparate in organizational placement and level, splitting intent and focus. These organizations need to *revitalize* their performance-improvement efforts.

CASE STUDY

Revitalization Case Study

The U.S. Navy Department of Medicine and Surgery initiated a system-wide performance-improvement program using Lean and Six Sigma in 2006. After approximately 12 months, it was determined that additional structure and oversight would be necessary to realize the results that an increased operational tempo and amplified budgetary demands required.

In 2007, a Continuous Process Improvement Program Office was established to execute the performance-improvement policies developed by Navy Medicine's executive leaders. The program office initiated efforts to develop a governance process to ensure that

CASE STUDY

performance-improvement guidance, support, and trained resources were available across the entire enterprise.

The first step was to contract for performance-improvement technical support. Master practitioners were assigned at each of the three Navy Medicine regions, as well as at the Navy Medicine Support Command at the program office. Later, an additional master practitioner was assigned to the Navy Department of Medicine and Surgery in Washington to provide support in policy development. The next step was to develop a deployment plan that would map out the initial phase of this integrated performance-improvement effort. A schedule for development of organic resources and delineation of the roles of the program office and regional performance-improvement resources were included.

The current Navy Medicine performance-improvement program is robust and realizing significant benefits literally around the world. Metrics are being reported monthly to the Navy Medicine executive leadership team as sigma scores, further reinforcing the cultural changes being realized within Navy Medicine.

Another organizational scenario is one that has been successful with performance-improvement efforts in the past, and now leadership wants to take the program to the next level—or *new heights*. In many ways, deployment in this type of organization is the most difficult. People become comfortable with the status quo—especially if it is meeting expectations.

While these descriptions alluded to organization-wide deployments, they also can be applied to division or department levels as well. In much the same way that an efficacious performance-improvement program must be robust across various deployment maturity levels, it also must be scalable to organizational size or even levels within an organization. While sustainment across an entire system historically has proven difficult, sound performance-improvement practices can be deployed within a single department or division—radiology, for example. In some cases, this limited deployment is applied as a pilot for a broader deployment in the future. While this method has worked in many organizations, it should be pursued with caution owing

CASE STUDY

New Heights Case Study

A small, single, not-for-profit hospital had been applying Lean methods successfully for several years. Most efforts were undertaken at a department level and were reported to the executive leadership team as successes. At some point, the chief financial officer (CFO) asked what was being done with the financial savings and increases in capacity that many projects had been reporting.

After a closer review of the reported savings, it was realized that several things were happening. First, in some cases, work was being shifted out of the process being improved and into a subsequent process. Another problem was revealed: Project outcomes were being based on local improvements, not system improvements. For example, an early step in a process was eliminated, and the time savings was extrapolated over the entire project. This resulted in a declared increase in capacity of 20 percent. What was not addressed was that the work simply moved more quickly to a complex step later in the process. At this step, the work built up because the later process had insufficient capacity. The net result was no true increase in Throughput. An integrated approach to performance improvement would have provided a better understanding of Constraints Management and taken the deployment to the next level.

to the high degree of interdependency between organizational entities within healthcare.

Many hospitals have deployed Lean and/or Six Sigma successfully. As their Lean Six Sigma deployments reach maturity, they have the opportunity to take their performance improvements to new heights by applying Constraints Management principles and tools. However, we recommend a phased approach for a controlled introduction of Constraints Management because major paradigm shifts required for its deployment can become overwhelming. Similar to getting into a hot tub, we do not simply jump in: Entering a hot tub begins by first easing in one's toes, then slowly the feet, followed by the legs until the entire body is submerged. Hence, introducing some tools and concepts of Constraints Management slowly and deliberately works well. This approach is described in detail in Chapter 7.

In addition to Constraints Management, incorporating systematic innovation tools such as Theory of Inventive Problem Solving (TRIZ), de Bono's thinking hats, and the Crawford slip method result in superior returns on investment for performance-improvement programs. Major corporations such as Intel, Pratt Whitney, ABB, Siemens, General Electric, and Caterpillar are already using them for breakthrough innovations as part of their performance-improvement programs. Deployment champions need to constantly remain current regarding the latest advances in performance-improvement methods, tools, and technologies to continuously improve their programs and adjust them as the competitive landscape changes and healthcare reform takes shape.

Four-Phase Integrated Performance-Improvement Approach

Success in performance improvement cannot be left to chance, nor can it be reactive in approach. It requires a structured, proactive approach to ensure both short-term success and long-term sustainability. Figure 3.3 shows our four-phase approach, called *system-based continuous-performance-improvement (SystemCPI)*, to deploying an integrated approach to performance improvement across virtually any organizational entity.

The leading performance-improvement methods across most industries are Lean, Six Sigma, and Constraints Management—which is based on the theory of constraints introduced by Goldratt. Each of these methods has complementary features, as shown in Figure 3.4.

Developed by NOVACES, LLC, the SystemCPI deployment roadmap shown in Figure 3.3 has incorporated the three methodologies in a single

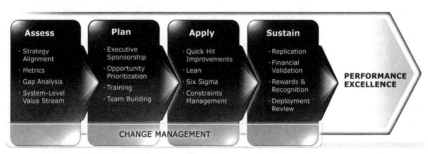

Figure 3.3 The four-phase performance-improvement approach.

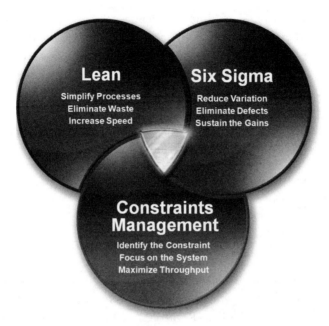

Figure 3.4 The complementary features of Lean, Six Sigma, and Constraints Management.

system-based continuous-performance-improvement deployment approach. By incorporating these best practices—both in the deployment approach itself and in the associated improvement efforts—the result is a truly integrated, sustainable approach.

An integrated performance-improvement approach that is focused on improving performance across an organization should bridge the gaps between an integration and a mix. Consider the analogy of a gallon of tinted paint and a load of mixed gravel. In the former, the component parts are indistinguishable, whereas in the latter, although the components form a single load, they still retain their distinct characteristics. Within an integrated approach to performance improvement, the degree to which the tools are truly integrated versus applied as independent entities is based on the deployment objectives. During the assess phase, Constraints Management thinking processes, system-level value stream analyses, and other traditional quality tools are integrated into a cohesive approach to identify high-impact improvement opportunities and ensure their alignment with the organization's strategy. On the other hand, in the apply phase, specific improvement methodologies may be blended. For example, a process-level value-stream analysis is used to identify capacity-constrained resources. Various methods are applied to address specific performance gaps. Applying these tools to improve performance will be addressed in Chapter 6.

An effective approach must look at the entire organization—a true systems approach—so that improvement opportunities can be identified end to end. An integrated performance-improvement approach recognizes five basic principles for a successful deployment:

▲ Involve executive leadership.
▲ Focus on execution.
▲ Be flexible in approach.
▲ Balance data and process knowledge.
▲ Drive to sustainment.

In addition to these overarching principles, it must address the two primary reasons for deployment failure: inappropriate project selection and limited executive involvement. Regardless of the approach used to deploy performance improvement, special attention must be paid to these challenges.

Figure 3.5 shows the roadmap of the entire integrated approach. This map will be used to focus the discussion as each component is discussed in detail throughout this book.

Assess

The assess step starts with a review of the organization's mission, vision, strategic goals, current process-improvement initiatives, and associated metrics. A triadic approach is used to identify performance gaps and other

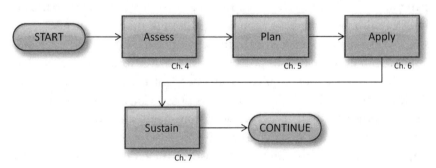

Figure 3.5 The integrated approach to performance improvement roadmap.

opportunities for improvement. This approach includes a strategic gap analysis to conduct organizational assessments and compare progress and performance against the goals and metrics established within the organization. A system constraint analysis then is conducted to identify various constraints that hinder performance, as well as to determine core drivers that serve as leverage points to focus improvement efforts. Lastly, a SystemVSA is conducted to identify the performance gaps in the system's core processes.

The expected outputs of these three analyses include

▲ A high-level diagram of the enterprise's core business processes
▲ An analysis of the gap between organizational goals and core process performance
▲ An assessment of the organization's level of performance-improvement maturity
▲ An assessment of the organization's change readiness
▲ An Intermediate Objectives (IO) map identifying the critical success factors and necessary conditions associated with organizational goal attainment
▲ A focused current reality tree (fCRT) or current reality tree (CRT) that identifies core drivers and core conflicts depending on the availability and desire of executives

As a result of these gap analysis and planning sessions, an *improvement opportunity worksheet* is developed. The worksheet lists improvement opportunities, the most likely improvement approach, links to strategic goals, core business processes, and core problem areas. Improvement opportunities are identified and listed, ranging from *quick hits* that can be implemented (most of the time) immediately to projects requiring the rigor of a Six Sigma project applying the define-measure-analyze-improve-control (DMAIC) methodology. The assess step is critical to overall deployment success. It establishes foundation and critical success factors that ensure that performance-improvement resources are directed at problems with the greatest global impact on the organization's goal.

Plan

The improvement opportunities identified in the assess phase are prioritized based on organizational impact and resource availability. A deployment plan is developed that details the path forward—identifying improvement opportunities, communications and training plans, as well as metrics to measure the overall success of the deployment. The executive leadership team is responsible for prioritizing and selecting the initial improvement opportunities to be addressed. Selection of the right projects is one of the key success factors in a performance-improvement deployment. This is followed by identification of a champion to sponsor each project and team members and delivery of just-in-time training for the selected improvement opportunities.

Fast-Tracking the Assess/Plan Phases

In an effort to quickly realize benefits from their deployment, a concentrated effort can be undertaken that accelerates progress from months to a few weeks. It literally jump-starts the entire deployment. Properly executed, this JumpStart compresses the timeline from kickoff through development of the deployment plan. This fast-track approach requires access to the executive leadership team over a two-week period. A significant amount of preparation is necessary prior to the start to ensure that materials are available for review and analysis. Members of the deployment team should be identified and be available to actively participate in the event. Most JumpStarts can be accomplished in two weeks. While JumpStarts lead to faster results, they require a higher level of concentrated commitment by the deploying organization than a traditional deployment. Figure 3.6 shows a generic two-week schedule.

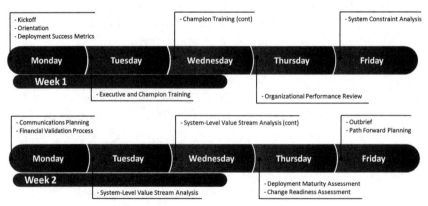

Figure 3.6 A typical JumpStart schedule.

Apply

This phase is about applying appropriate performance-improvement tools and getting the desired results. Depending on the nature of the improvement opportunities, tools and methodologies are used in the appropriate sequence to get the desired results. These include quick hit improvements, process value stream analyses (ProcessVSAs), rapid improvement workshops, Six Sigma DMAIC projects, Constraints Management, and even revisiting the strategic planning process. At the start of all process-improvement projects, teams should examine past and ongoing process-improvement projects to determine which of those projects—their methods, findings, recommendations, and results—can be leveraged in the current effort being undertaken.

Sustain

This phase includes identification of replication opportunities within the organization. Each project team reviews its respective project for replication opportunities in order to maximize return on investment. Finally, the financial and operational impact of the deployment is reviewed. The contributions of individual projects then are compared against the overall cost of the deployment. A control plan ensures that any deviation from the anticipated path toward the future state is recognized and addressed immediately and appropriately. This prevents a regression to the mean or a return to the "way it's always been done."

The people side of sustainment is critical: It is the people who drive the improvement and ensure its success. If their efforts are not recognized, the deployment will fail eventually, as countless others did. Hence it is critical to sustain the motivation of the participants with an effective reward and recognition program.

Deployment success metrics and program alignment with strategy should be reviewed regularly, at least annually. In a constantly changing environment, the sails of a performance-improvement deployment must be constantly trimmed to capture the changing winds and propel the deployment forward.

Conclusion

The structured approach to deploying performance improvement through healthcare organizations is critical. Issues relating to required deliverables, leadership and staff involvement, and timeline must be addressed, and even methodologic decisions must be made. These activities and decisions should be clearly documented in a deployment plan and endorsed by the executive leadership team. This chapter provided a recommended structure based on the NOVACES, LLC, deployment approach known as SystemCPI. Subsequent chapters will describe the application of an integrated toolset to deploy a robust yet rigorous performance-improvement program beginning with the first step, assess, in Chapter 4.

CHAPTER 4

Assessment

"There is one art of which man should be master, the art of reflection."

—SAMUEL TAYLOR COLERIDGE,
ENGLISH ROMANTIC POET AND PHILOSOPHER

The assess phase is the most crucial phase in performance-improvement deployments. And yet it is the one that receives the least attention in many such deployments. The work done builds the foundation by which performance improvement is deployed across the organization. Lack of leadership commitment and involvement is a critical point of failure for any performance-improvement initiative. In this phase, commitment by the executive leadership team is essential. The steps built into the assess phase not only contribute to the technical aspects of how performance improvement will be implemented, but they are also designed to drive executive commitment.

An organization's mission, vision, and value statements are the foundation for its strategic planning, performance assessment, and improvement activities. All members of the deployment team should review and understand these statements. These objectives will be validated during this phase. They will seldom change, but the discussion will bring them to the forefront and ensure understanding and alignment. The deployment team also will conduct a structured review of available performance-related information to identify and better understand gaps between the organization's performance and its mission and strategy.

The assess phase consists of a three-part, or triadic, approach to identifying performance gaps across the organization, as shown in Figure 4.1. These three assessments, strategic gap analysis, system-level value stream analysis, and system constraint analysis, do the following:

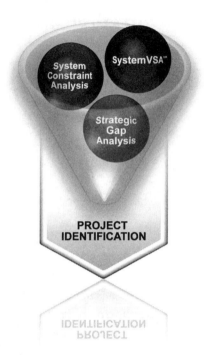

Figure 4.1 The three assessments.

▲ Provide insight into organizational goals and identify performance gaps through reviews of existing metrics and other information sources
▲ Identify measures of success for core processes
▲ Distinguish critical success factors and conditions necessary for goal attainment
▲ Pinpoint core problem areas that, when addressed, provide the most leverage toward goal attainment

Strategic Gap Analysis

The *strategic gap analysis* is accomplished as the first event of the triadic approach. It is usually conducted first because it can provide the deployment team with information regarding existing performance gaps that will facilitate both the system-level value stream analysis and the system constraint analysis. In many cases, this is the first time that information,

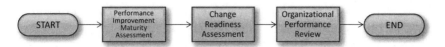

Figure 4.2   Strategic gap analysis roadmap.

data, or metrics about the organization undergoing the JumpStart are available for review. The strategic gap analysis includes two organizational assessments and an organizational performance review. The first step is to assess the organization's current level of performance-improvement maturity and its readiness for change. Figure 4.2 shows the strategic gap analysis roadmap.

Performance-Improvement Maturity Assessment

This assessment quantifies an organization's progress through the performance-improvement maturity model. As demonstrated in Figure 4.3, progress through the four phases of a performance-improvement deployment correlates with progress toward self-sufficiency.

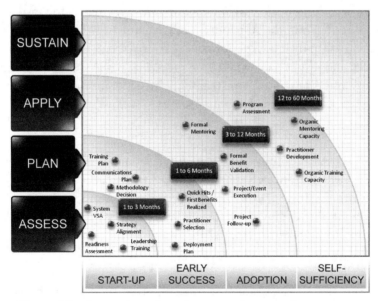

Figure 4.3   System-based continuous-performance-improvement (SystemCPI) maturity model.

▲ The phases of the deployment are contained in individual boxes on the *y* axis to communicate the four distinct phases.

▲ The overlap in the timeline connotes that a fixed timeline is not possible. It depends on many variables within each organization.

▲ Organizations do not move from one stage into the next but transition through them with overlap.

Program maturity is a common metric for assessing an organization's progress toward program goals. In "A Study of the Relationships in Financial Performance, Organization Size, Business Classification, and Program Maturity of Six Sigma Systems," Diane J. Olson found that there was no significant relationship between program maturity and years of implementation. This is evidence of the wide variation in time anticipated to attain advanced maturity levels.

Completion of the phase deliverables or outputs establishes the correlation between the deployment and organizational maturity. In the performance-improvement maturity model shown earlier, critical deliverables are delineated within their respective phase. Each phase of performance-improvement maturity is treated as a distinct construct with multiple questions for each.

A discussion on the development approach as well as the instrument itself is available in the Appendix. The instrument is made available for readers to use in their own performance-improvement deployment. Sharing feedback and results data would be appreciated so that we may continually validate and improve the instrument. Instructions for providing the feedback are also included in the Appendix.

Delivery

The performance-improvement maturity assessment is administered to the senior leadership team early in the deployment. In most cases, the assessment is conducted during the JumpStart. It can be administered periodically throughout the deployment to validate progress, either manually or electronically, whichever is more appropriate for the organization.

Reporting

The results of the assessment can be reported on a chart similar to a barometer or a stacked bar chart. As the cumulative score increases, advancement through the maturity levels is indicated. A review of multiple deployments at various stages and with varying levels of success results in recognition of the breakpoints that differentiate the maturity of performance-improvement deployments. Since the scale is 1 to 5 with 16 questions, the lowest possible score is 16, whereas the highest is 80. The breakpoints across the maturity levels are as follows:

▲ 16 to 50 = startup
▲ 51 to 60 = early success
▲ 61 to 70 = adoption
▲ 71 to 80 = self-sufficiency

Individual construct scores also should be displayed. This demonstrates progress along the model. An organization in early success would score the majority of points in the first two constructs and then taper off in the final two. During normal maturation of an organization, one would expect the cumulative score to rise increasingly owing to the contribution of higher adaptation and self-sufficiency scores. When an organization's cumulative score indicates a lower maturity level, yet the individual construct scores are somewhat evenly spaced across all levels, as in Figure 4.4, this is indicative of an allopathic approach to process improvement.

Much like the allopathic approach to medicine in the post–Civil War era, the allopathic approach applies science—but not necessarily the

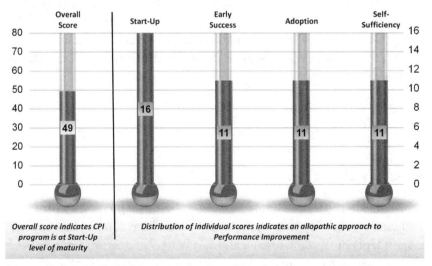

Figure 4.4 Maturity assessment: allopathic approach example.

scientific method. During most of the nineteenth century, if a patient did not die and recovered, it generally was assumed that whatever treatment was given must have been responsible for the cure. The practice of allopathy prevailed so long precisely because, despite being drained of their blood and poisoned with highly toxic drugs, many patients did, in fact, recover from serious infectious diseases such as yellow fever and cholera. The lesson to be learned is that, like patients who recover naturally from deadly diseases thanks to their own vitality and despite receiving the harmful allopathic treatments, so might quality or performance gaps improve even when the improvement approach lacks rigor or fails to address root causes. Organizations and people do what is necessary to succeed. While these disjointed and potentially harmful efforts may be locally or initially successful, they do not necessarily lead to sustainability or reproducibility. A scattershot approach sometimes may hit the mark, but surely there must be a better way.

Change-Readiness Assessment

Readiness for change is a prerequisite to successful change. We have developed a *performance-improvement-focused change-readiness assessment survey*. It is based on a review of available literature as well as discussions with both change-management and continuous-performance-improvement practitioners. While there is much discussion about the potential constructs that can be incorporated into a change-readiness assessment, it is agreed that the inclusion of the following constructs supports both the face and content validity of the assessment. The assessment includes five constructs of change readiness:

▲ Communications
▲ Culture
▲ Leadership
▲ Organization
▲ Skills readiness

While there has been limited success in developing a robust instrument that addresses all constructs, the assessment's item content should focus respondents on specific organizational change. In *Medical Care Research and Review*, Bryan Weiner and colleagues found that this limitation has a

CASE STUDY

Maturity Assessment

A medium-sized not-for-profit hospital system wanted to assess its performance-improvement maturity. As part of the JumpStart, the performance-improvement maturity assessment was administered.

The system's overall score for performance-improvement maturity on the assessment tool was 37. This placed the deployment in startup. Based on an anecdotal assessment, this result was well within the anticipated range. As seen in Figure 4.5, the scores from the individual constructs indicate a reactive and somewhat unstructured approach to performance improvement that is commonplace but especially prevalent in industries that have a history of identifying quality or performance gaps and initiating independent corrective actions.

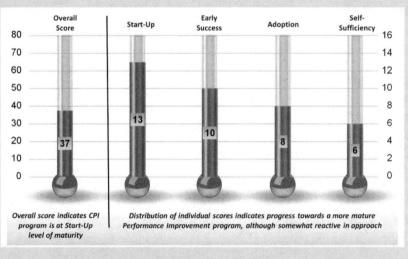

Figure 4.5 An example of a maturity assessment.

negative impacts on the applicability of a single instrument across a broad range of changes. The assessment applied during the performance-improvement deployment balances general constructs with a focus on improving performance.

A baseline assessment is administered early in the assess phase. An action plan should be developed based on the results. During the sustain phase, the instrument should be administered a second time. This comparison will provide a measure of change-management success.

A discussion on the development approach, as well as the instrument itself, is available in the Appendix. The instrument is made available for readers to use in their own performance-improvement deployments. Sharing feedback and results data would be appreciated so that we may continually validate and improve the instrument. Instructions for providing the feedback are also included in the Appendix.

Delivery

The change-readiness assessment should be administered to a broad sample of the organization population. It can be done manually or electronically, whichever is more appropriate for the organization.

Scoring

The assessment is scored as follows: Each individual item receives the following score based on the selected level of agreement:

▲ Strongly disagree = 1
▲ Disagree = 2
▲ Neutral = 3
▲ Agree = 4
▲ Strongly agree = 5

The scores then are averaged for each construct (i.e., communications, culture, leadership, organization, and skills readiness) and displayed graphically. Each construct is to be addressed separately based on the respective scoring range.

Reporting

The results of the change-readiness assessment are reported as a chart that allows both a comparison across the five constructs and the goal of a score of 4.0. Each axis represents a separate construct. The mean score for that construct should be displayed prominently. A score of 4.0 is considered acceptable across all constructs. An example of a reporting chart is given in Figure 4.6.

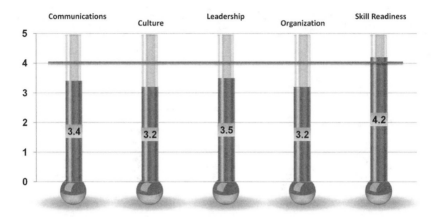

Figure 4.6 Change-readiness assessment.

The findings are presented with comments and/or recommendations associated with each construct score. The results of the assessment should be reviewed by the deployment team. While the scores themselves are somewhat telling, their linkage to specific observations and anecdotes will make the findings and subsequent recommendations more impactful.

CASE STUDY

Change Readiness Assessment

A medium-sized not-for-profit hospital system decided to implement an integrated approach to performance improvement across the system. As part of the JumpStart, the change-readiness assessment was administered. Its findings are presented in Figure 4.7.

Communications were assessed as fair, but blockage continued to occur. Somewhere in the organization, open communications were being rerouted or stifled. Many employees sensed that more was going on than they were being told. They were eager to hear more, especially because it affected their work. They needed more information to better serve their patients. It came, but in spurts rather than a continuous flow. The key here is to discover where the obstruction lies and to unblock

CASE STUDY

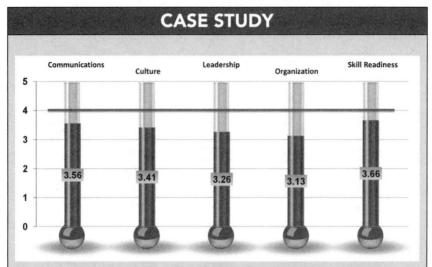

Figure 4.7 Change-readiness assessment: case study.

clogged communications. Using all available resources is recommended to totally remove the clogs in addition to opening communication channels. This serves to open a whole new world for employees.

Organizational silos limited the free flow of information between divisions and departments. Accountability and responsibility were novel concepts and therefore suspect. The reward and recognition system had improved, but occasionally punishments were more visible than positive incentives. Employees wanted to see their tasks and assignments as important to the success of the organization. Leaders and supervisors would have to drive the changes needed in order to improve recognition and tear down remaining silos.

While there was a vision of the future, to the employees, it appeared fuzzy and lacking substance. The employees wanted to trust their leaders but found it difficult. Performance improvement had become a catch phrase rather than a business strategy. The employees knew the hospital could do better in serving its patients. During times of significant change, they sought clarity as to the organization's direction and focus. Only occasionally did they find it. The key here was to reemphasize the vision and ask, "Where is the organization headed?" "How will it get there?" and "Is performance improvement a cornerstone for the organization?"

CASE STUDY

Being those closest to the problems, employees believed that their knowledge of the organization, its customers, and its services was being wasted. They had heard about the success of cross-functional teams, and they wanted to use them in their own work areas. They wanted to be "team members" and experience actual decision making. In their eyes, accomplishing this would contribute to making their departments and their hospital system a "high performer."

While the employees sensed some teamwork initially, they feared it was not enough. They viewed their skills as good but not great. They wanted to improve the effectiveness of their work areas and the organization as a whole. They knew that they could do better, but they felt that they may have lacked the necessary knowledge or training. They needed two things simultaneously: increased access to training and a sharper focus on teamwork. With these, their self-confidence would grow quickly.

Organizational Performance Review

An *organizational performance review* is conducted to identify improvement opportunities and core problem areas through review of existing data and results of inspections and certification reviews by regulatory or accrediting agencies. The review is conducted with the deployment team and during work sessions with the executive leadership team. The findings should be compiled and included in the deployment plan. Some examples of the type of information reviewed are addressed below.

▲ **Patient satisfaction survey.** Loyal patients are a hospital's best asset and can be more powerful than any marketing campaign. Measuring patient satisfaction can be a key indicator of overall organizational success. Patient satisfaction measurement can be conducted internally or through external providers who can rank performance against peers.

▲ **Hospital Survey on Patient Safety Culture.** In 2004, the Agency for Healthcare Research and Quality (AHRQ) released the Hospital Survey on Patient Safety Culture, a staff survey designed to help hospitals assess the culture of safety in their institutions. Since then, hundreds of hospitals across the United States and internationally have implemented the survey.

▲ **Joint Commission Periodic Performance Review.** The Periodic Performance Review is a compliance assessment tool designed to help healthcare organizations to continuously monitor performance and performance-improvement activities. The review provides the framework for continuous standards compliance and focuses on the critical systems and processes that affect patient care and safety.

▲ **Center for Medicare and Medicaid Services (CMS) core measures.** Quality measures are used to gauge how well an entity provides care to its patients. Measures are based on scientific evidence and can reflect guidelines, standards of care, or practice parameters. A quality measure converts medical information from patient records into a rate or percentage that allows facilities to assess their performance.

▲ **Healthcare Effectiveness Data and Information Set (HEDIS).** The Healthcare Effectiveness Data and Information Set (HEDIS) is a tool used by more than 90 percent of America's health plans to measure performance on important dimensions of care and service.

▲ **National Database of Nursing Quality Indicators.** The National Database of Nursing Quality Indicators is a proprietary database of the American Nurses Association. The database collects and evaluates unit-specific, nurse-sensitive data from hospitals in the United States.

▲ **Internal metrics.** Virtually all healthcare organizations have established some set of internal metrics to assist leadership in managing the business. While the content of these measurement systems varies greatly, most include information from the previously cited sources.

Reporting

The organization performance review is documented using the Improvement Opportunity Worksheet. A sample template of an organizational performance review appears in Figure 4.8. The worksheet should be adjusted as necessary for the specific engagement and is used to document all improvement opportunities identified during the early stage of the deployment until a more sophisticated portfolio management system is developed or adopted.

			Alignment with									Criteria Ranking			
			Strategic Goals			Areas			Core Processes			.xx	.xx	.xx	
Project Idea	Champion	Champion Trained (Y/N)	Strategic Goal #1	Strategic Goal #2	Strategic Goal #3	Core Driver #1	Core Driver #2	Core Driver #3	Core Process #1	Core Process #2	Core Process #3	Selection Criteria #1	Selection Criteria #2	Selection Criteria #3	Ranking

Criteria weights

Figure 4.8 Improvement opportunity worksheet.

CASE STUDY

Organization Performance Review

A large not-for-profit healthcare system deployed the integrated approach to performance improvement. The primary objectives for the deployment were to improve the patient experience and reduce costs.

As a part of the deployment, a JumpStart was conducted, including the organization performance review portion of strategic gap analysis. The deployment team gathered performance data from hospital departments and divisions. In the absence of a balanced scorecard, more than 100 disjointed internal and external measures of organizational performance were reviewed and analyzed.

Sources included the CMS core measures, the results of the Press Ganey Patient Satisfaction and Culture of Safety surveys, a state department of health audit and Joint Commission periodic performance review findings, and HEDIS and other quality indicators. Current levels of performance were assessed relative to requirements, targets, and strategic objectives. When a gap existed, a process owner was identified and data were collected to quantify the gap. These performance-improvement opportunities were added to the performance-improvement opportunity portfolio to be prioritized and, if selected, chartered as performance-improvement projects or events.

For example, a presurvey Joint Commission preparation review had identified egress to be a problem. Means of egress is the second most

CASE STUDY

common citation issued by the Joint Commission, with 50 percent of hospitals noncompliant, as reported by Evan Sweeney in his article, "'Means of Egress' Remains as a Top Joint Commission Citation." Linen carts and other equipment blocked fire doors and exits and clogged corridors. This citation was noted on a previous survey, increasing the urgency of the issue and the prioritization score for 5S rapid improvement workshop opportunities related to the problem. A system-wide 5S event was scheduled. Of Japanese origin, 5S is a Lean method to create and maintain an organized work environment.

The communications team publicized the event using multiple channels and venues. Lean experts presented a brief 5S training module to participating departments. Because the event was early in the deployment, the deployment champion noted, "I'll be happy if we charter five events." More than eighty 5S events over the course of three days resulted in the elimination of more than 20 tons of trash. Storerooms were cleaned and organized, and materials and equipment were stored according to Lean principles, such as point of use, kitting, and visual management. Linen carts were reconfigured, and hallways and exits were cleared. There were no egress-related citations when the Joint Commission survey occurred several months after the event.

System-Level Value-Stream Analysis

Introduced in Chapter 3, a roadmap of a *system-level value-stream analysis (SystemVSA)* appears in Figure 4.9. A SystemVSA is intended to accomplish three goals for the organization:

▲ Identify the core business processes and decompose those processes to a point where data can be collected, gaps identified, and action taken.

▲ Ensure that core business processes are aligned with the organization's mission, vision, and values.

▲ Focus improvement efforts on the critical processes directly supporting the strategic goals.

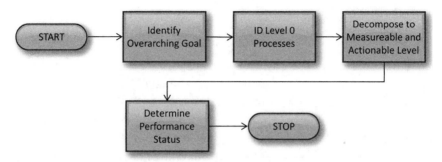

Figure 4.9 System-level value-stream analysis roadmap.

The event generally is facilitated by an experienced performance-improvement practitioner with the organization's executive leaders participating as team members. The practitioner should have experience in working with executives because active participation by the executive leadership team is critical. The SystemVSA generally occurs as a single event over one to two days (including data collection and gap analysis). Prior to the event, the practitioner should become familiar with available data sources within the organization. This is largely accomplished through conduct of the organization performance review prior to the SystemVSA.

In addition to establishing the foundation for future improvement efforts, the results of the SystemVSA can be used to provide input for the development of an ongoing performance dashboard, as addressed in Chapter 6. As the performance gaps are closed, managers can monitor certain metrics to ensure that improvement efforts are progressing and that objectives are being met. The value of monitoring certain key metrics rather than monitoring *all* metrics is to focus efforts on the gaps that are most critical or linked most directly with strategic imperatives. Additionally, since the identified core processes exist at a higher level, the knowledge gleaned can be used to drive future strategic planning efforts.

The SystemVSA, when employed properly, enables senior leaders to focus more strategically and lower-level leaders to identify and sponsor more tactically relevant projects. The major steps of the SystemVSA are discussed next.

Initiating the SystemVSA

Identification and Documentation of Core (Level 0) Processes

Level 0 processes are the core processes (enabling processes are addressed below) that contribute directly to organizational success. While the term *core process* is used, the intent is to encourage the executive leadership team to identify and focus initial efforts on the processes that are the reasons the organization is in business. The value or level of contribution of a process should not be dictated by an arbitrary distinction but by the value attributed to it within the organizational context. This may result in a knowledge-based organization (such as a health system) considering a process for staff retention or employee development to be a core process because it makes sense strategically despite its more common categorization as an enabling process.

While the focus of the SystemVSA is on core business processes, this does not obviate the potential to apply it to enabling or supporting processes. While alignment of improvement opportunities with core processes often results in the highest impact on organizational goals, improvements to enabling processes also may have a positive impact on overall goal attainment—albeit in a less direct manner.

If it is determined that identification and decomposition of enabling processes are appropriate, they can be conducted as part of the SystemVSA event or may be accomplished separately. In many instances, enabling processes are less strategic in nature, and decomposition may be accomplished at a level below the executive leadership team—accounts payable, for example (assuming that it is identified as an enabling process), may be decomposed by a team from the finance department. It is important to realize that what is considered an enabling process in one organization may be considered a core process in another organization.

Identification of Metrics and/or Subordinate-Level Processes

In many cases, level 0 processes are not measurable. If measurement is possible at level 0, then it is not necessary to decompose the process further. If measurement is not possible, then decomposing the process into subordinate processes is necessary to identify metrics by which process capability can be quantified. If there is a *performance gap* (a difference between current performance and targets or objectives), an opportunity for improvement has been identified. In a SystemVSA, processes are identified by process name only. Process steps are not identified. As each process is identified, two questions are asked:

▲ Can the process performance be measured at this level?
▲ Is a performance gap actionable at this level?

If the answer to both questions is "Yes," then the right level of decomposition has been reached. In identifying how the process can be measured, the use of existing metrics is preferable to the development of new ones. If no metrics are available or gaps are not actionable at level 0, then level 1, level 2—or the next-lower-level—processes must be identified to quantify process performance and identify potential gaps.

An example of how an overall SystemVSA is mapped in a hospital is shown in Figure 4.10. It is best when displayed hierarchically beginning with the level 0 processes and decomposing downward to the level where data are available. The figure shows this aggregated presentation. As a means to further clarify the individual components of the SystemVSA, each vertical segment can be documented separately.

Identification of Gaps

In many cases, while the gaps or opportunities may have been identified in the strategic gap analysis, they were not necessarily linked to actionable processes. Additionally, acceptable levels of performance—specification limits—may not have been defined. Data should be reviewed to quantify gaps versus acceptable levels—thereby identifying improvement opportunities. During the SystemVSA, a process owner should be identified for each process at the lowest level of decomposition. The process owner, in conjunction with other attendees, estimates the efficacy of the process. When possible, efficacy should be defined in term of time, cost, and quality. Figure 4.11 shows a process information form that is used to capture this information.

Data Collection and Validation

While an initial assessment of process efficacy is accomplished during the event, the process owner then must validate that estimate. Data collection and validation of the lowest levels of the SystemVSA are accomplished subsequent to the event. Time is included in the JumpStart schedule to identify and collect available data. Metrics at the levels associated with a

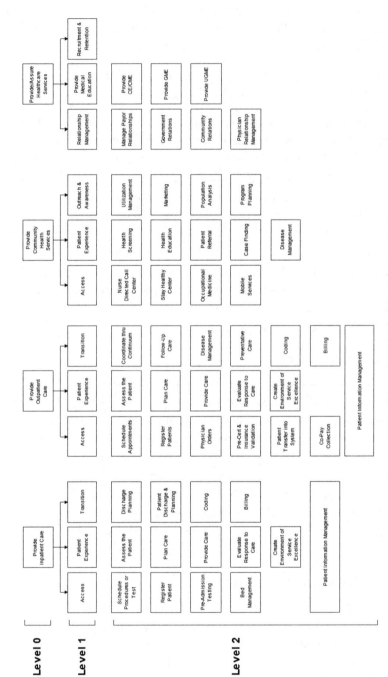

Figure 4.10 SystemVSA example for a hospital.

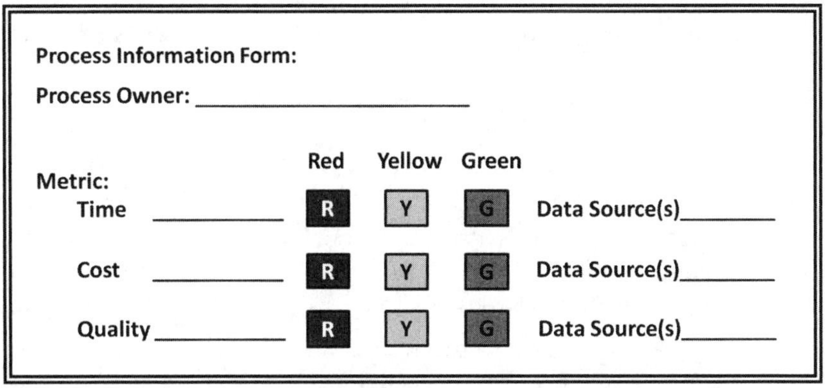

Figure 4.11   Process information form.

SystemVSA typically are dashboard or stoplight indicators representing a roll-up of multiple subordinate indicators. Metrics reported to senior leadership generally reflect core capability as defined by the organization.

It is important that this data collection is distinguished from data collection associated with a Six Sigma project. Statistical certainty is not the primary objective. The intent of the SystemVSA is to gain an understanding of performance gaps, and the goal is to identify opportunities for improvement.

SystemVSA Outputs

There are two distinct sets of outputs from the SystemVSA. The first is the graphic documentation of the SystemVSA itself, which is a hierarchical view of the decomposed levels of the VSA down to the point where measurement is possible and actionable. The second is the identification of potential performance gaps and their inclusion in the Improvement Opportunity Worksheet.

System Constraint Analysis

The *system constraint analysis* applies a portion of Constraints Management thinking processes, as illustrated in the roadmap in Figure 4.12. The underlying premise is that pure process-related gaps generally are identified through other analyses (e.g., SystemVSA or strategic gap analysis). The focus

CASE STUDY

System-Level Value Stream Analysis

A SystemVSA was conducted during the assess phase of a JumpStart at a not-for-profit healthcare system. The system is comprised of two large medical centers, one of which is a university-affiliated teaching hospital, and a network of primary- and specialty-care clinics, and community and long-term care centers. Initially, the executive leadership team struggled to distinguish between departmental silos and core processes, and the SystemVSA closely resembled the organizational chart. This is common in an organization new to more sophisticated performance-improvement methods. A product family perspective was needed to help the team to identify the essential core processes through which the system delivers value to its customers.

As a product of the analysis, level 0 (the highest level) core processes including "Provide community health services and community outreach" in addition to "Provide inpatient care" and "Provide outpatient care" were identified. Each level 0 process then was decomposed into level 1 core processes. Level 1 processes included high-level processes such as "Provide medical education," "Ensure access," and "Transition of care." The team identified processes with increasing granularity until it could be verified that some data or metrics existed by which to evaluate process capability in terms of cost, time, and quality and that the performance gaps were actionable.

"Transition of care" had been identified as a level 1 process for both "Inpatient care" and "Outpatient care." Leadership had identified a "Fully integrated system" as the corporate vision of the organization. Analysis of the data revealed that opportunities for improving "Transition of care" processes existed in each dimension of process capability. Admission, transfer, and discharge took too long. Care was not coordinated adequately across the continuum. Errors and omissions occurred. Performance related to existing measurement systems was inadequate.

Specific performance-improvement opportunities related to "Transition of care" were identified and prioritized. Several performance-

CASE STUDY

improvement projects were chartered and completed, each clearly linked via the SystemVSA to organizational strategy. These projects and events have transformed "Transition of care" processes such as admission, discharge, transfer, follow-up, medication reconciliation, and care management. Process performance is being monitored and reported through control plans and scorecards. The cumulative impact of these efforts has moved the dial on a level 0 core process identified as a strategic imperative by executive leadership.

of the system constraint analysis is the identification of system constraints as well as core drivers to focus improvement efforts. Application of the *Intermediate Objectives (IO) map* serves as the primary vehicle to start the analysis.

Intermediate Objectives (IO) Map

As introduced in Chapter 2, the *IO map* begins with identification of the overarching goal and the critical success factors or terminal outcomes required to meet that goal. The critical success factors then are followed by identification of the necessary conditions or key outcomes from activities required to make the critical success factors happen. An example for an outpatient service is shown in Figure 4.13.

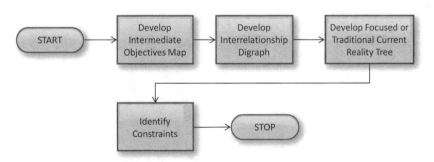

Figure 4.12 System constraints analysis roadmap.

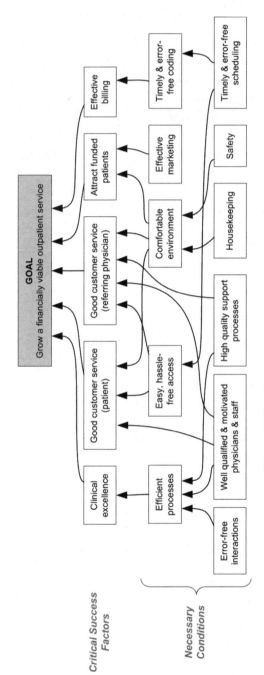

Figure 4.13 IO map: outpatient service example.

Focused Current Reality Tree (fCRT)

The *focused current reality tree* (fCRT) is used to identify core drivers. This is extremely useful when prioritizing and selecting improvement projects.

There are several approaches to generating an fCRT, but we have found that the following process is highly effective and can be accomplished comparatively quickly. Completion time is a critical factor because executives are frugal with their time. Through tight facilitation and expert tool application, some of these tasks can be accomplished quickly—thereby exceeding expectations.

Using the IO map as a source document, brainstorm the undesirable effects (UDEs) that can result when the critical success factors identified in the IO map are not realized. A sufficient number of UDEs should be generated so that they can be evaluated and refined to a list of the critical eight to ten items, although the number varies. The list can be reduced through multivoting or other consensus-generating tools.

Once the UDEs have been refined to the critical few, an *interrelationship digraph*, as described by Nancy R. Tague in her book, *The Quality Toolbox*, can be applied to identify potential core problems or focus areas. The UDE with the most "out" arrows signifies a strong influence/causing impact—and should be considered a *core problem area*. The rule of thumb is that the number of core problem areas should be limited to no more than three.

The completed interrelationship digraph, as shown in Figure 4.14, then is used to develop the fCRT. The core problem areas are listed at the bottom, and then the hierarchical nature of the graphic shows the linkages from the core problem areas through secondary problems (UDEs) to the goal. The intent is to demonstrate improvement activities within core drivers that have the broadest impact on the goal because they will affect multiple secondary problems. Not all problems brainstormed—or even identified through multivoting—will be included in the fCRT. These items can be considered as independent improvement opportunities and included on the Improvement Opportunity Worksheet. Each improvement opportunity should be reviewed for linkage to the core drivers identified via the fCRT, which is shown in Figure 4.15.

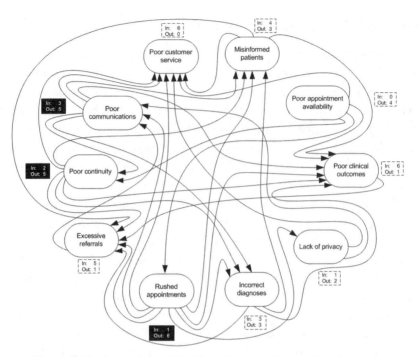

Figure 4.14 Interrelationship digraph: outpatient services example.

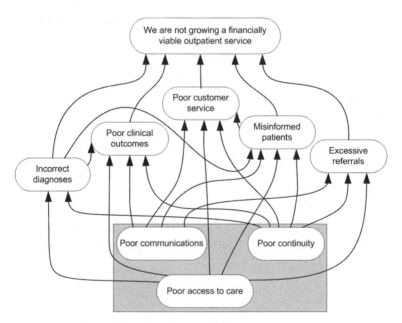

Figure 4.15 fCRT: outpatient services example.

Identify System Constraint

The workshop participants then are asked which of these critical success factors or resulting UDEs are negatively affected by constraints. A champion should be identified for each constraint. Once identified, these constraints are addressed in the deployment plan and outbrief. They are then included on the Improvement Opportunity Worksheet. Policy or market constraints generally require more direct leadership action than the typical improvement opportunities listed. In some cases, policy constraints can be mitigated as relatively simple *quick hits*. In others, more complex leadership action is required. In many of the latter instances, adjustments to the strategic plan may be necessary.

CASE STUDY

System Constraint

A medium-sized hospital was in a quandary. It faced an apparent market constraint—having the resources and capacity to treat far more patients than were passing through its doors. A CRT from Constraints Management's thinking processes was constructed and analyzed to verify that the constraint of the hospital was in the market and to gain deeper insight into its root cause. While the CRT was quite large, as can be seen in Figure 4.16, it nonetheless proved extremely useful in revealing one of the core drivers for the market constraint, as well as an associated policy constraint.

Under the conditions of a market constraint, paid resources who were ready, willing, and able to treat patients were sitting idle. What is surprising is that the market constraint was based largely on a policy of the hospital to not accept an insurance provider that covers a large percentage of the population. This decision was made based on calculations using the hospital's cost accounting system. The hospital's financial management team could get a more clear picture by adopting direct costing (or variable costing) decision support. Such a support system prevents patient rejection when the patient's insurance will cover the totally variable costs associated with the patient's treatment when there is free capacity.

CASE STUDY

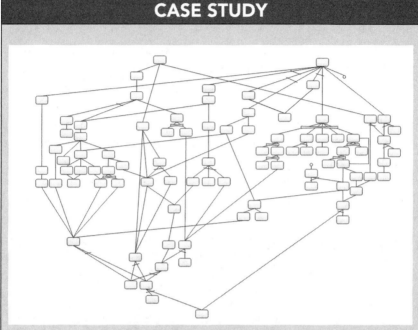

Figure 4.16   CRT example.

Beyond cost accounting methods driving the hospital to reject paying customers in conditions of a market constraint, the CRT established a core driver. It had been intended to be a general-purpose hospital with a wide range of services when it was founded, and the insurance environment at the time was conducive to making such an operation financially viable. However, since the insurance conditions changed significantly, the decision was made to discontinue providing coverage to patients with that specific insurance. This decision, in turn, reduced the hospital's patient volume significantly.

With a new strategy, the hospital would have decided to focus its efforts along a particular medical specialty. Therefore, it would not have invested in some of the equipment that was unnecessary to provide coverage in those services. As a result, this would have allowed a reduction in fixed costs. If the hospital avoided investing in equipment unrelated to its specialties, it could have attained more specialized

CASE STUDY

technology and recruited specialist doctors, increasing its differentiation and expanding overall patient Throughput significantly. In brief, the system constraint analysis uncovered some surprising results. At its core, it revealed that the hospital needed to revisit its strategy in the new market conditions, and the CRT showed insights on what to change.

Conclusion

The foundation to be laid during the assess phase is often neglected entirely or given cursory attention at best. It is neither glamorous nor does it provide tangible results such as realized in the apply phase. However, as with the foundation of a house, if this phase is not done well, the house ultimately will collapse under the rigors of the environment in which it stands.

The importance of leadership commitment and involvement has been stressed as a critical factor in the failure of any performance-improvement deployment. In the assess phase, commitment by the executive leadership team is ensured. The assess phase is the time to set the expectations for deployment and establish ownership by the executive leadership team. Once the current state has been assessed, planning can be pursued in the next phase. The importance of planning, what to plan, and how to plan it follow in Chapter 5.

Planning for Deployment

"A goal without a plan is just a wish."

—LARRY ELDER, RADIO TALK SHOW HOST

This chapter discusses the key components of planning a performance-improvement program deployment. The improvement opportunities identified in the assess phase are prioritized based on organizational impact and then scheduled based on resource availability. A deployment plan is developed that details the way forward for improvement opportunities, communication and training plans, and metrics to measure the overall success of the deployment. Team members are identified, and delivery of just-in-time training for the selected improvement opportunities is accomplished.

Why Plan?

No one denies that planning is necessary, but how it is done is open to a broad range of approaches and opinions. Some contend that Frederick Taylor's seminal work on scientific management is the basis of all business planning. In the book, *Business Planning*, Darren O'Connor describes a direct linkage from the basic tenets of management science to business planning:

▲ Analysis
▲ Decomposition
▲ Efficiency

These three tenets were incorporated into the early strategic planning processes developed by the U.S. military and later incorporated into the corporate world. They are equally applicable in healthcare. One way to view planning is that the future will only become reality by envisioning it, preparing for it, and executing it, as Rick Page observed in the book, *Hope Is Not a Strategy*. In many instances—especially in healthcare—the gap is in operational planning. An effective plan must be what Andrew Green calls a "blueprint for action" in *An Introduction to Health Planning for Developing Health Systems*.

Creating this "blueprint for action" requires the commitment, time, and effort of providers. By investing these in planning, time is taken away from patient care, managing staff, balancing budgets, and an endless list of other responsibilities described by William Sibbald and Thomas Massaro in *The Business of Critical Care: A Textbook for Clinicians Who Manage Special Care Units*.

Competition between these critical components of leadership's day-to-day duties is one of the primary reasons performance-improvement deployments fail. Without executive involvement and commitment, there can be no plan. Without a plan, action lacks focus and structure. Without focus and structure, true success cannot be achieved.

Deploying performance improvement in healthcare organizations is a complex and time-consuming process. It requires a certain level of planning to ensure success. When deploying a successful performance-improvement program, it is important that things be done in a certain order. While somewhat flexible, the order will ensure that the deployment has a solid foundation.

A great way to envision the order is to look at the sequence shown in the progression along the *performance-improvement maturity model*. Completing these steps requires oversight and active management.

Timeline

Once again, using the *performance-improvement maturity model* as a basis, Figure 5.1 shows a high-level deployment timeline. As can be seen readily, there is significant variation across deployments. Factors affecting the timeline include organization size, geographic dispersion, leadership involvement, and local leadership autonomy. Organizations should balance taking the time to do it right with the realization that the longer it takes to start improving performance, the longer performance will need improvement.

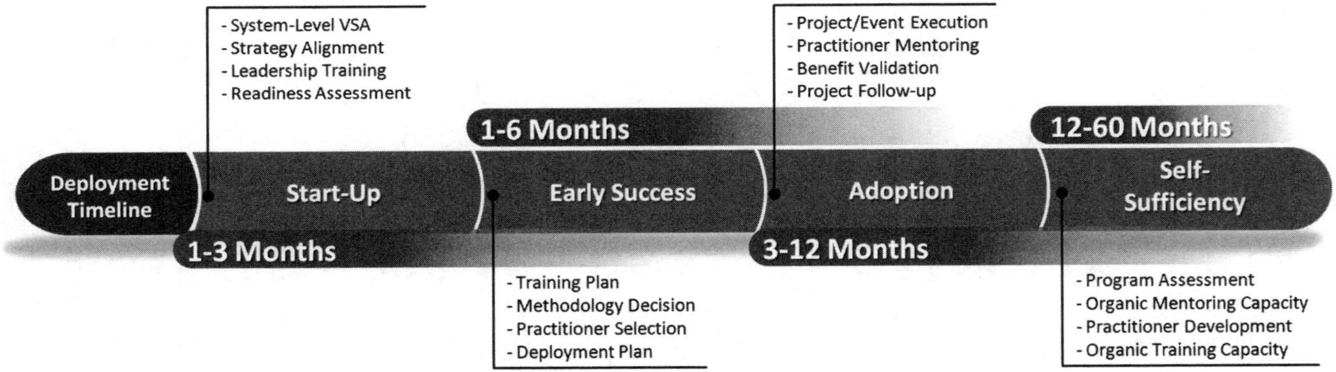

Figure 5.1 Performance-improvement maturity model.

Deployment Timeline

Start-Up — 1-3 Months
- System-Level VSA
- Strategy Alignment
- Leadership Training
- Readiness Assessment

Early Success — 1-6 Months
- Training Plan
- Methodology Decision
- Practitioner Selection
- Deployment Plan

Adoption — 3-12 Months
- Project/Event Execution
- Practitioner Mentoring
- Benefit Validation
- Project Follow-up

Self-Sufficiency — 12-60 Months
- Program Assessment
- Organic Mentoring Capacity
- Practitioner Development
- Organic Training Capacity

Deployment Metrics

Whenever a healthcare organization is committing itself to deploying a performance-improvement program, leadership must codify and articulate the reasons for the initiative. Deployment metrics must be developed to determine if these reasons are being addressed and the deployment is progressing successfully. Whenever these metrics are not meeting the target, course corrections can be made before the long-term success of the initiative is compromised.

Identifying the Correct Measures

Deployment metrics typically are segregated into two or three categories. The first two types are pivotal to understanding how a deployment is progressing toward objectives and achieving anticipated benefits and the desired changes.

The first category of metrics tends to be based on volumes. These are often referred to as *density metrics*. The second category is *business metrics*, which are used to show the overall efficacy of the deployment or its impact on the business. The final category is *sustainment metrics*, which measure how well the deployment is progressing toward self-sustainment.

Density Metrics

Density metrics are most often the easiest to define, and they measure how well the organization is embracing the new initiative into the operational fabric of the enterprise. The typical measures are broken down into several categories for measuring progress of the implementation. Density metrics might include

▲ Training volume
▲ Divisional/departmental participation
▲ Number of projects

Once density metrics have been identified, operational definitions must be articulated that ensure consistency in data collection. Even the most intuitive measures—such as the definition of *projects*—can have vastly different interpretations within the organization.

While these metrics tend to be somewhat shallow and risk becoming an end in themselves, they are extremely important and must be collected.

Ultimately, they should become part of the larger set of deployment metrics and not viewed as the only measures of success.

Business Metrics

The second category of metrics, commonly referred to as *business metrics*, links the customers' needs with the health of the business. Every enterprise has business metrics, and typically, they have matured to the point where most employees recognize them and understand their definitions. These business metrics are those typically demonstrated on periodic or annual reports or are used by leadership to determine overall progress toward organizational goal attainment. Business metrics can be developed and applied at any level within an organization.

Moving the dial on these metrics is the reason that the vast majority of organizations deploy performance improvement. In healthcare, examples of critical business metrics are length of stay and rates of infection. Connecting the initiative to the business goals is important to demonstrate that the efforts of the deployment have made a difference in the enterprise's performance and goals. Leadership should set the expectation that a successful deployment of the system will make a positive impact on the business metrics. This direction will align the resources and efforts toward the goal of improving those outcomes. Through deployment planning, projects and events are selected and chartered that are aligned with activities that affect business metrics.

Sustainment Metrics

Density metrics were the first measurements that were developed and carefully defined in the early phases of a performance-improvement deployment. Next, the overall efficacy of the deployment was linked to business metrics, many of which had been defined previously. The third and final category of metrics is commonly called *sustainment metrics*. Sustainment metrics examine assimilation of the new culture and capabilities that have resulted from the deployment. Most deployments require external assistance and expertise. These can be viewed as one-time events. The duration of these expenses should be addressed in the deployment plan, and a timeline should be attached.

External resources are often necessary to *prime the pump*. Consultants may be used for program design, initial training, mentoring, and organic capability development. The costs associated with this support should decrease over time, whereas the internal capability should increase. Sustainment metrics might include

▲ Number of certified practitioners (multiple levels)
▲ Training conducted with internal resources
▲ Deployment costs
▲ Mentoring hours

Sustainment metrics are deployed by leadership with an eye toward the organizational culture and capability of the entire organization. Periodic application of the change-readiness and maturity assessments is another means by which to measure an organization's culture and performance-improvement progress.

Proper development of deployment success metrics is critical. While the metrics are often adjusted throughout a deployment, the initial set should be developed early. Given this level of flexibility and adjustability, many deployments focus initially on the density metrics. While this is common and poses no real threat to overall success, it poses a risk of over-emphasizing volumes, such as number of people trained and number of projects, rather than progression toward identification or development of business and sustainment metrics.

Given the possibility that metric development could stall at the density level, careful attention should be paid to outlining a success metric development timeline in the deployment plan. The assignment of specific responsibility for the ongoing identification and development is critical for deployment success.

Governance

Successful performance-improvement programs cannot run without governance. But governance does not equal bureaucracy. In the book, *Physician Practice Management*, Stephen Wagner uses a diagram to describe group practice governance. Modified, this graphic is equally applicable to performance-improvement program governance.

Figure 5.2 demonstrates that governance is based primarily on the strategic goals of the healthcare organization, tempered by the organizational culture. The means by which gaps are identified, as well as the efforts

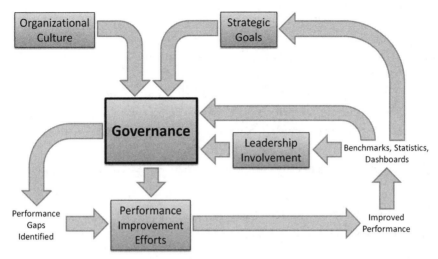

Figure 5.2 Performance-improvement program governance.

to close the gaps, must be managed and channeled. Feedback then is provided to leadership, which reinforces its continued involvement and drives refinement of the organizational strategies.

Governance of a healthcare organization's performance-improvement program can take different forms. It can exist within existing quality management or performance-improvement departments, or a new program management office (PMO) can be formed to lead the effort. Wherever placed, a single entity should manage performance-improvement efforts across the organization.

As addressed previously, a deployment team is formed during the initial stages of the deployment. It should include team members with the following roles or their representatives:

▲ Deployment champion
▲ Patient care leadership (chief nursing office, nurse manager, physician leader, etc.)
▲ Communications (public affairs, community relations, etc.)
▲ Human resources/organizational development
▲ Finance
▲ Executive leadership team

A team member from human resources/organizational development advises on matters relating to position descriptions, organizational culture, and change management. Someone in a finance role assists in the development of the benefit-validation criteria/process.

The level of focus that a dedicated PMO can provide the deployment will greatly enhance the likelihood of overall deployment success. The organizational placement, structure, and formation of the PMO need to be determined as early as possible in the plan phase because the life cycle of the deployment team generally ends once the deployment plan is published.

Who Are Performance-Improvement Practitioners?

Performance-improvement practitioners apply various performance-improvement tools and techniques to close or mitigate performance gaps throughout an organization. All practitioners are change agents—evangelists for quality and business results—whose passion for excellence motivates and energizes individuals and teams.

The names and levels of performance-improvement practitioners vary greatly across methodologies. When considering Lean, Six Sigma, and Constraints Management, it is easy to see why something as simple as what to call the practitioner can be a barrier to integrating the methods.

Lean

While Lean principles are intended to be applied by all employees at all levels of an organization, the term *Lean sensei* is used to describe advanced Lean practitioners. The word *sensei* is used to show respect to someone who has achieved a certain level of mastery in an art form, skill, or discipline. In their book, *Lean Thinking*, Womack and Jones recommend that those seeking to achieve organizational effectiveness should seek out a Lean sensei.

Six Sigma

There are three primary levels of Six Sigma practitioner: *Master black belts* are fully trained practitioners who have a more "managerial" role, in that they often are responsible for all Six Sigma work done in a particular area or function. Typical duties include selection, training, and mentoring of black belts, project selection or approval, and review of projects completed. They are expected to have a deeper technical knowledge of the tools as well as other soft skills. *Black belts* are fully trained practitioners normally assigned Six Sigma projects on a full-time basis and are responsible for mentoring green belts. *Green belts* are not trained in advanced statistical methods and are assigned Six Sigma projects in addition to their normal duties. The training received and projects led by green belts vary the most across organizations.

Constraints Management

In his business novel, *The Goal*, Eliyahu Goldratt introduced Jonah as a character. Jonah served as an advisor to the main character, Alex, and helped him to break down a complex system to figure out the constraint in the system and understand its functioning. Since then, the term *Jonah* has evolved as a thinking processes practitioner. The Theory of Constraints International Certification Organization (TOCICO) certifies Constraints Management practitioners using more descriptive terms: *practitioner*, *implementer*, and *academic*. As described by the TOCICO,

- ▲ Practitioners are responsible for planning and/or execution as well as continuous improvement of TOC-related applications that have already been implemented at a company.
- ▲ Implementers are responsible for the design and implementation of the new rules and related logistical systems, processes, and metrics of one or more of the TOC applications.
- ▲ Academics are responsible for teaching TOC applications to practitioners and/or implementers.

To promote use of the appropriate methodology in support of goal attainment and to avoid advocating one approach over another, the simple terms *practitioner* and *advanced practitioner* will be used.

Advanced Practitioners

An advanced practitioner is the most capable and diverse of performance-improvement practitioners. In general, advanced practitioners are successful practitioners who have demonstrated exceptional leadership and technical skills, have completed projects successfully, and have proven their ability to teach and mentor other performance-improvement practitioners. Further, they exhibit the desire and aptitude to master advanced concepts and skills and are strong candidates for future leadership roles in the business. The advanced practitioner demonstrates mastery-level expertise across a variety of performance-improvement methodologies. An advanced practitioner translates performance-improvement philosophies and methods for understanding and application across the boundaries of position, function, profession, and industry. Advanced practitioners are also change agents with the business acumen, political savvy, and communications skills necessary to institutionalize performance improvement.

What Do Advanced Practitioners Do?

A unique blend of attributes and competencies is required to fulfill the complex role of the advanced practitioner effectively. The advanced practitioner is a technical leader by virtue of his or her expertise and experience related to leading performance-improvement methodologies. The depth and breadth of knowledge of the advanced practitioner allow for the effective use of tools and methods to solve complex problems and achieve strategic objectives. This includes leading complex, especially high-risk, and enterprise-level projects. The advanced practitioner employs interpersonal and change-management skills to engage stakeholders at every level of the organization and forge partnerships with business leaders to remove barriers, minimize resistance to change, and resolve conflicts.

Building and facilitating teams to complete performance-improvement projects and accomplish program objectives, advanced practitioners ensure that team success is recognized, rewarded, and celebrated. The advanced practitioner identifies and communicates opportunities for improvement and recognizes and disseminates best practices. Advanced practitioners act as project managers, maintaining the momentum of projects and events to achieve measurable business results within expected time frames. Their role includes assisting other practitioners to

▲ Define and scope projects
▲ Estimate and validate project savings
▲ Evaluate the integrity of measurement systems

▲ Perform complex statistical analyses
▲ Establish project milestones and tollgate review schedules
▲ Communicate results to key stakeholders

As a coach, the advanced practitioner fosters the integration of generally existing skills into a new context. Coaching includes helping leaders to adapt their skills to leading in a performance-improvement-focused environment. As a mentor, the advanced practitioner nurtures the development of less experienced practitioners. This guidance generally is accomplished within the context of performance-improvement projects or events. The advanced practitioner evaluates the competencies and attributes of the individual, identifies and mitigates skills gaps, and creates opportunities for development specifically directed toward aiding and encouraging practitioners to achieve their full potential.

Where Do Advanced Practitioners Come From?

Advanced practitioners generally are practitioners who demonstrate mastery of technical, management, and leadership skills. Some common requirements for advancement include training materials development, training and mentoring other practitioners, leading enterprise- or business-level performance-improvement events and projects, and leading deployment support activities such as the development of templates, reports, and metrics. The advanced practitioner also must possess essential "soft" skills, including change management, networking and influencing, coaching, mentoring, and conflict resolution. The most appropriate means of obtaining and using this valuable resource depends on the goals and objectives of the deployment as well as the organization's strategy and capacity to achieve them. If the objective is to change the culture of the organization and establish a world-class, enterprise-wide performance-improvement program, the best solution likely will include the development of advanced practitioners from within. This requires commitment and capacity in terms of time, people, and other resources to achieve such an ambitious target.

An organization whose objective is to use selected performance-improvement tools and methods to execute a specific strategy or solve a discrete set of problems may not have a sufficiently compelling business case, near-term capacity, or level of commitment to make such an investment. In the absence of sufficient organic knowledge of performance-improvement methodologies and deployment strategies, the experience and expertise of a consultant are indispensable. This is especially true during the early phases of a deployment, when critical decisions must be made related to policy and infrastructure, roles and responsibilities, training requirements, reward and recognition structures, program measurement, and program governance.

As described below, an advanced practitioner is neither born nor created but is developed. This development requires time and conditions conducive to experiential learning. The apprentice-journeyman-master approach is the optimal model. A newly graduated medical doctor has a good understanding of anatomy and physiology but does not become a surgeon without first completing internship and residency. There are three options for obtaining advanced practitioner services: rent, buy, or grow, as shown in Figure 5.3.

Rent One

During the startup phase of a deployment, most successful deployments use the services of an external performance-improvement consultant. If the strategy is to achieve performance-improvement self-sufficiency, a consultant will work closely with the client organization to design a deploy-

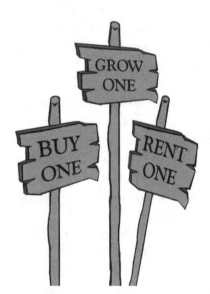

Figure 5.3 Options for advanced practitioners.

ment with this goal in mind. After the initial deployment, there are advantages and disadvantages associated with using consultants. The advantage is the immediate availability of their expertise and experience in the short term. The disadvantage is that even the most customer-focused consultant is not a part of the organizational culture. While imperative during the initial phases of the deployment, their outside-in view may have a negative impact on or slow the organic growth of a performance-improvement culture. Employee perception that the company is not investing in its own people may, in time, hinder deployment efforts and stunt cultural transformation. For small healthcare organizations with fewer than 100 employees, renting an advanced practitioner is usually the most cost-effective option.

Buy One

On the surface, it could appear that hiring advanced practitioners to kick-start a performance-improvement deployment at the outset would save time and money. This does not take into consideration the time, expense, and risk involved in recruiting and hiring any new employee. The standards for performance-improvement practitioner training, development, and certification vary broadly. Practitioners are a product of their training and experience. Individual distinctions may or may not match a particular healthcare organization's deployment objectives. If there are any key competency gaps that need to be closed, training for the new employee would require a considerable investment up front. If the decision is made to hire an advanced practitioner, it is imperative that the position requirements be specific, comprehensive, and clearly defined. Hiring managers who interview candidates will need to know the appropriate questions to ask candidates and the correct answers to those questions.

Recruiting and hiring practitioners without organic knowledge of requisite competencies and attributes can result in hiring the wrong person for the role or incorrectly defining the role to be filled. Even if the new hire possesses all the competencies and attributes of an advanced practitioner, orientation of any new employee takes time and costs money. The advantages of internal advanced practitioners include ownership and knowledge of internal culture. It would take some time before a newly hired practitioner could achieve this level of assimilation into the organization. It would be especially difficult for the newly hired practitioner to fulfill the role of change agent. Finally, hiring an advanced practitioner does nothing to mitigate the many risks associated with contracting performance-improvement expertise. Therefore, many organizations use the services of consultants through the initial phases of the deployment, and some take advantage of the consultant's experience and expertise in the hiring process.

Grow One

A long-term solution is to internalize performance-improvement expertise by developing this critical resource from within. Growing talent from within begins with selecting the right people to become practitioners. This selection requires dedication of the best and brightest to performance improvement. Filling practitioner positions with the "expired and expendable" is a sure path to deployment failure. Without the strong guidance of an advanced practitioner, organic development is all but impossible. When attempting to grow talent from within, it is often necessary to contract with an external source to mentor apprentice practitioners. As with any employee selection and development process, specific selection criteria that include characteristics predictive of success should considered.

Practitioner Selection

Second only to leadership involvement, the selection of performance-improvement practitioners is the most important people issue of a deployment. *Rath & Strong's Six Sigma Leadership Handbook* recounts that David Cote, president and CEO of Honeywell International, said that all black belts and master black belts would be selected from employees who had been identified as highly promotable and that the time spent as practitioners would be viewed as a career accelerator.

While Mr. Cote was discussing a Six Sigma deployment in manufacturing and not a more robust integrated performance-improvement deployment in healthcare, his comments are certainly applicable. Practitioners, especially those selected to full-time roles or who will be expected to progress to an advanced level, should be the best that the organization has to offer. They should have the capability and self-confidence to influence, negotiate, and resolve conflicts to reach consensus. Performance-improvement practitioners must have an understanding of not just the organization but also its business processes and how they work together across multiple divisions and operations. They should have an appreciation of the expectations of all key stakeholders, always be mindful of the customer, and constantly consider the impact of decisions during all stages of a project.

It should be understood that performance-improvement practitioners are expected to be change agents, challenging traditional ways of doing business and cutting through red tape to make substantial improvements. Their communications skills and their ability to discuss ideas and recommendations with senior leadership within the organization—their ability to stand in front of the senior leaders and talk about their projects—should be among the best in the organization. They should be able to communicate concepts, manage relationships, and collaborate with others.

In addition to these interpersonal skills, they should exhibit exceptional writing, math, and statistical analysis skills. Computer literacy is extremely important. They should have experience with Microsoft Office products, specifically Excel and PowerPoint for basic data analysis and presentations. They may be expected to learn new software programs to perform advanced statistical analysis and process mapping. They may have to access online tools, libraries, and databases for research.

Individuals selected to become performance-improvement practitioners should be performing at a high level in their current job and display agility and the ability to work effectively under pressure, as well as the potential to rise to the highest levels of leadership in the organization.

Practitioner Development

While many healthcare organizations realize great success with a performance-improvement deployment, some fail to attain the levels of success that they had hoped for. The reasons for these less than optimal results are numerous. Previously, two prevalent causes were cited: lack of executive involvement and poor project selection. Another factor is failing to develop practitioners.

The apprentice-journeyman-master developmental model for performance-improvement practitioners is widely accepted. In the classroom, the subject matter, pace, and timing of the knowledge transfer are largely controlled by the curriculum. From the initial application in the guilds of Europe, the apprentice-journeyman-master model has served many professions. Electricians, pipefitters, and plumbers are obvious examples in that they maintain the same naming conventions. In academia today, the same approach is used, but it is known by different names. A thesis or dissertation needed to get an academic degree is examined by "master practitioners"—professors—in much the same manner as a journeyman cabinetmaker may have produced a masterpiece—not in the artistic sense but as in "master piece"—for review by a master cabinetmaker in order to be accepted as a master himself or herself.

Another modern example of the apprentice-journeyman-master model is the career path of the professional engineer. Although the requirements vary slightly from state to state, in general, to obtain a professional engineering license, one must graduate with a bachelor of science in engineering degree from an accredited college or university, pass the engineer-in-training (engineer intern) exam, work in the discipline for at least four years under a licensed professional engineer, and then pass the professional engineers' exam to obtain a professional engineering license.

To illustrate the model in healthcare, this approach is analogous to the transition from medical student to intern to resident to physician. After the student completes a predetermined amount of didactic learning, the intern begins to practice under the guidance of a mentor; then, based on readiness, the resident begins mentoring less experienced interns; and finally, the resident makes the transition to a fully independent practitioner. While not attempting to compare the complexity or level of knowledge of an advanced performance-improvement practitioner with a fully qualified physician, the developmental path is nonetheless similar.

The role of the mentor becomes critical in the development of advanced practitioners. This model has been applied since pre–industrial revolution craftsmen took in apprentices and developed them to become masters in their own right. Many mentoring programs are a pull, or reactive, system, where the mentor becomes involved at the request of the practitioner, or protégé. This pull system puts the responsibility on the new practitioner for determining what is needed and when. Recognizing that the new practitioners don't know what they don't know, how can they be expected to solicit help on the right topics at the right time? This has a direct, negative impact on long-term program success. Successful development of a performance-improvement practitioner requires a push system, in which the master practitioner mentor determines the skills needed, provides training and guidance as needed, and assesses the developing capabilities of the protégé.

Mentoring: An Art and a Science

Mentoring must be viewed as a combination of science and art. *Science* refers to the infrastructure, tools, and metrics associated with knowledge transfer. *Art* refers to the actual relationship between the mentor and the protégé. Both these aspects need to be addressed in order to set the conditions for a successful mentoring program.

The science of mentoring should start with a clearly articulated statement on the desired goal. Prioritization of mentoring goals should be driven by the strategic, operational, and tactical goals of the performance-improvement deployment. Science includes the development of standards and procedures to govern the mentoring process that address such subjects as the frequency and duration of mentoring sessions, the environment, and the required tasks that must be performed. An effective means of standardizing the process is through the development of mentoring guides and process documentation. Use of such documents gives the mentor a framework through which to accomplish the organizational objectives set out in a deployment plan.

The art of mentoring, much like the more traditional use of the term, is somewhat difficult to define and traditionally varies from mentor to mentor. It is driven by the fact that there will always be some variability in the conduct of mentoring activities that depend on personality, experience, behaviors, and respect. The reality is that mentoring cannot be forced on an individual. It is common practice in performance-improvement deployments to assign mentors to protégés to assist in their development. The truth is that to be effective, mentoring cannot be forced on an individual. A person must want to be mentored. What is often found is that practitioners first must buy into the mentor as a person before they will buy into being mentored. In establishing a successful mentoring environment, the first critical step is to establish a relationship based on trust and credibility. In truly effective mentoring relationships, the person being mentored selects the person by whom he or she would like to be mentored. Unfortunately, if this were a standard practice in large-scale deployments, the more experienced and popular mentors would end up with a larger caseload, whereas other advanced practitioners would end up with fewer protégés. This is the reason that mentors are assigned protégés in typical deployments.

Achieving the right balance between the science and art of mentoring without losing the focus on the overall goal of achieving results is the key. Having advanced practitioners burdened with a large number of administrative tasks associated with project tracking ends up taking away from the time available for knowledge transfer or coaching of candidates. On the other hand, having little to no administrative tasks limits advanced practitioners' interaction with the organization. What is the right mix? As with most organization-wide change efforts, this depends on the objectives and focus of the business. The answer is the balance between art and science, typified in Figure 5.4, and it must evolve as the healthcare organization evolves.

Mentoring traditionally has been viewed as a means to an end and focuses primarily on knowledge transfer between the experienced mentor and the practitioner. To drive true results, the mentor must be invested in or have a stake in the process. How much vested interest does the mentor have in the protégé completing the project successfully? Does the mentor see his or her role as simply a conduit for knowledge transfer or as actually pushing protégés to close projects and realize results?

The mentor must realize that project closure and results are goals of the deployment. With this realization, the responsibility, accountability, and

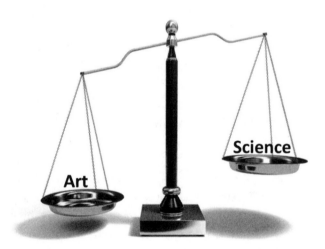

Figure 5-4   Mentoring—balancing art and science.

authority of the mentors must be aligned. Deployments where mentors and protégés are held equally responsible for results tend to have higher closure rates and shorter cycle times. Benefits are realized sooner. Why does this practice lead to results? Because the mentor typically has more experience of what it takes to close a project successfully and is more knowledgeable regarding how to use team-building and influencing skills to overcome roadblocks and drive projects to success. Holding both the mentor and the protégé responsible ensures that there is *accountability* of all concerned.

Mentoring Drives Results

The objective of any performance-improvement effort is results. A look at some mentoring programs from a value-stream analysis (VSA) perspective defines mentoring as an administrative task. With any process, there needs to be administration. Performance-improvement administrative tasks should take a subordinate role to driving project closure, results, and knowledge transfer. There are many automated project tracking and management systems available to aid in maintaining situational awareness of projects, results, and financial benefits. Some claim that they can replace the role of the mentor in the execution of projects. These systems may be used to decrease reliance on mentors when the focus of the senior practitioner or mentor is transferred from project closure to maintenance of the database to ensure that the most relevant information is available. This practice removes responsibility for project management from the practitioner, which is a development need. A danger in any deployment is creating a bureaucracy around project visibility that causes the practitioner to spend more time maintaining program status tracking and completing templates than actually implementing solutions and obtaining results. When this environment exists, a performance-improvement effort creates the very bureaucracy it was chartered to eliminate.

The solution is to apply sound performance-improvement principles to the deployment and continually assess how much time is spent by whom, maintaining the tracking and management database versus driving project closure, results, and knowledge transfer.

In most performance-improvement training venues, soft skills such as effective communications, influence without authority, conflict management, and obtaining the commitment from critical stakeholders are considered mere respite from more technical subjects, such as advanced statistics. A study in the United Kingdom by Jiju Antony and colleagues found that the ability to communicate effectively was the most essential skill for a performance-improvement practitioner.

While deployment failures tend to be caused by lack of leadership involvement and poor project selection, individual projects fail because the stakeholders were not included or their buy-in was not achieved. It is somewhat contradictory that while a lack of soft skills tends to adversely affect project success more than a lack of knowledge of technical topics, the proportion of time spent developing them is significantly less. This occurs, to some degree, because it is assumed that employees selected for practitioner training already possess soft skills. The classroom is certainly the place where foundations for communications, influence, conflict management, and team dynamics can begin, but mastery of these skills must be developed in a mentoring environment.

The fundamentals of change management apply internally to a performance-improvement deployment. Changes in economic environments, customer requirements, and even culture and leadership drive healthcare organizations in different directions from year to year. Some of the changes in focus are dramatic, and some are more evolutionary. As the business continues to change focus, application of the organization's performance-improvement efforts must change with it.

To keep a performance-improvement effort alive and a viable part of a business, the focus must constantly change to keep pace with business needs. Good mentors are an essential part of this equation. But the mentors may need to be "retooled" occasionally to drive the program in the new direction in which the healthcare organization is headed. This may mean training advanced practitioners and mentors in new or additional best practice methodologies that are applicable to new objectives. During the course of a deployment, it may be necessary to require mentors to undertake projects personally so that they can build their experience base and hone their skills, stepping temporarily back into the journeyman role. An investment in continued training for advanced practitioners will be compounded through their mentoring and have a multiplier effect throughout the organization.

Goals for and approaches to mentoring must be addressed early in the deployment and then reexamined as the deployment matures. Mentoring must be a driving force in both accelerating project closure and refocusing efforts to align with business needs and objectives. Making mentoring about more than just teaching tools is a critical consideration in both individual project success and overall deployment success.

Practitioner Utilization

The issue of practitioner utilization is essential and should be addressed early in the deployment. Specific factors must be addressed, such as organizational alignment, full-time versus part-time status, and expectations regarding the number of improvement efforts to be completed. Personnel matters such as career paths and succession plans also should be determined. The dilemma is synthesized in the conflict cloud appearing in Figure 5.5.

Deployment Communications

"The problem with communication is the illusion that it has occurred."
—GEORGE BERNARD SHAW, IRISH PLAYWRIGHT

Communication is a process. A *deployment communication plan* documents the process by which information regarding the deployment will be disseminated. The plan is updated and revised as the deployment develops, milestones are met, and obstacles are encountered. Initially, communication

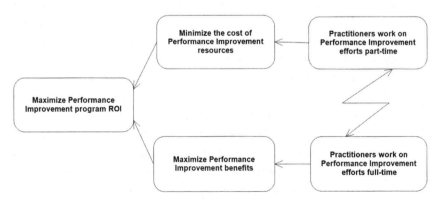

Figure 5.5 Conflict cloud: practitioner utilization.

is top-down. Leadership involvement is one of the factors strongly correlated with performance-improvement deployment success. Support for an initiative, such as a performance-improvement deployment intended to transform the culture of the organization, must be evidenced by leadership action and consistent, clear, continuous communication. A strong, engaged leader delivers a powerful message.

Development of a deployment communication plan is an essential activity that must occur no later than the early phases of development of a performance-improvement program. According to John Kotter's *Harvard Business Review* article, "Leading Change," 70 percent of reengineering endeavors fail. A communication plan is not only an influencing strategy but also a change-management strategy that can determine the success or failure of a performance-improvement deployment. As Carolyn Pexton writes in her article, "Communication Strategies for Six Sigma Initiatives," one of the lessons learned reported by healthcare providers actively applying Six Sigma is "Overcommunicate by a factor of 1,000!"

Proactive communication is critical to manage expectations and resistance to change. Communication related to a performance-improvement deployment must occur well before the first practitioner is trained or the first project or event is chartered. The very latest that a communication plan should be launched, at least in a preliminary format, is when a decision has been made to launch a performance-improvement program. This proactive plan communicates executive leadership's vision and strategies, thereby benefiting all levels of the organization. Change is the inevitable result of a performance-improvement initiative, whether it is a success or not. Planning for change and developing a strategy to manage responses and resistance to it require an effective and efficient communication plan. The best means of communicating leadership's commitment to a deployment is through their actions.

Communication is not an event. Important messages must be heard over and over again. Communication is iterative and ongoing. However, an event or events can be used to implement part of a communication plan. One of the best examples of the format and content, brevity, and impact of the initial message from leadership to the organization was delivered by CEO Jack Welch to General Electric (GE) employees in 1995. Watching the short video was mandatory for every GE employee. Welch's simple statement that Six Sigma would be the most important priority for the company for the next five years set the stage for one of the most successful performance-improvement deployments ever achieved. Communication across GE didn't stop there. Several years later, when Six Sigma had become ingrained in the company, messages about Six Sigma and then Lean Six Sigma were everywhere. No one could be a part of the GE culture and *not* know how performance improvement was defined by the company.

The deployment team is selected based on their knowledge and influence within the organization. The team should include representatives from the communication and/or marketing departments. These subject-matter experts are familiar with the communication processes, venues, and vehicles used to disseminate information across all levels of the organization, including customers and suppliers beyond the bricks and mortar of the organization. An evaluation of the effectiveness and reach of the organization's communication infrastructure is part of the assess phase of deployment planning. If it is found to be inadequate, improving this critical infrastructure element should be considered as an early focus for performance-improvement endeavors.

Once the deployment team has been provided with sufficient orientation and training to understand their role and the basics of the deployment strategy, as well as the tools and methods to be launched, team members will have the organic ability to develop and deploy the plan. The initial plan is best crafted under the guidance of an advanced performance-improvement practitioner because extensive knowledge of performance-improvement tools and methods that include change management is needed. While the deployment team exists as a temporary entity, the communication plan is ongoing and will be the means by which progress toward deployment objectives and milestones and the success and celebrations will be publicized. As process owners of ongoing communication, it is especially important that those who will *own* the plan going forward are involved in its development and understand the elements and importance of it.

Communication Plan

An effective communication plan provides information needed in the right format, via the right vehicle, in the right venue, at the right time, and producing the right results. In the vacuum created by the absence of such a plan, rumor, speculation, doubt, and cynicism will fill the gap. Resistance to change will increase, and the likelihood of a successful deployment will diminish quickly. An efficient communication plan provides all the information needed and nothing more.

The communication plan developed to support a performance-improvement deployment is much like any other strategic communication plan: It is crafted based on the results of a stakeholder analysis. Conducted during the assess phase of a performance-improvement deployment, a *stakeholder analysis* identifies stakeholders as any person, persons, department, or entity affected by or having the potential to affect the deployment. Each stakeholder then is evaluated in terms of his or her source of power and how he or she will be affected and/or have the potential to affect the success or failure of the deployment. Their current level of support for the deployment is evaluated. Analysis of the gap between the current and necessary levels of support guides the development of a communication strategy directed toward each stakeholder. The plan lists the actions to be taken to implement the strategy, moving or maintaining the stakeholder's position on the "support" end of the scale, and closing the gap.

All stakeholder groups are target audiences for the deployment communication strategy. The target audience determines the *what, when, where*, and *how* of a communication plan. Efficiencies of scale can be achieved by recycling such elements as the definition of performance improvement, the business rationale for pursuing it, and how the performance-improvement program will be deployed. But the perspective, needs, and anticipated response of each target audience should be considered when developing the plan.

Who

In healthcare, communication strategy would differ by degree from slightly to significantly depending on *who* the target audience is—physicians, nurses, other professional and operational staff, or department managers. For example, the content of a two-hour awareness session for medical executive leadership would differ significantly from that of an introduction to the performance-improvement deployment for practitioner candidates.

The careful planning of communications is especially important when targeting physician stakeholders in healthcare. The chief medical officer or some representative of the medical executive committee should be involved in deployment planning from the beginning. Creating the consensus and buy-in of physicians never should be left to chance or deferred. Physicians can become the greatest obstacles to or the most powerful proponents of a performance-improvement deployment. Which they become largely depends on the effectiveness of the communication plan. As critical stakeholders, their influence cannot be overestimated. Creating support for performance improvement from physicians is one of the most difficult challenges in healthcare. Making them an integral part of the solution is critical to diminishing resistance. Creating physician evangelists who will become formal and informal champions of the deployment is possible. In fact, it is essential if true transformation of healthcare is to occur. This change cannot be achieved without an effective communication plan that addresses physician interests and concerns.

Nurse stakeholders represent another key segment and target audience that requires careful, customized communication planning. Nurses will not usually demonstrate resistance to performance-improvement endeavors, at least overtly. The active and enthusiastic engagement of nurses is critical to the success of any healthcare performance-improvement deployment. Quality management and quality improvement are not new concepts to nurses. They are familiar with quality tools and methods used to meet accreditation and regulatory requirements, such as root cause analysis and the find-organize-clarify-understand-select–plan-do-check-act (FOCUS-PDCA) strategy. The communication plan must recognize the quality efforts already undertaken by nurses and describe how a performance-improvement deployment will augment the work that has been and is being done.

Nurses have received mixed messages about such performance-improvement methods. To them, such methods frequently mean *more work*. This is often true because nurses are called on to perform tasks such as data collection without any real understanding of what the data will be used for. In other instances, they associate performance-improvement efforts with reducing staff. When viewed together, such an approach can be seen as *more work with fewer people*. This is a message, whether intended or articulated, that inevitably will result in substantial resistance from nurses. As staffing cuts have deepened and nurse workloads have increased, anything that is perceived as adding to the burden already shouldered by nurses or diverting time from patient care will be viewed with distrust. Nurses are wary of change. Disconnects between nurse managers and their staff are common, and trust is a rare commodity. As with most caregivers, nurses understand the *business* of healthcare, but it is not their primary concern. The communication plan for nurses must make a clear connection between performance improvement and patient care. Demonstrating how the performance-improvement program will improve patient safety, satisfaction, and quality of care is the key to engaging nurses.

What

The *what* of communications evolves as the deployment matures. Initially, the message is focused toward removing barriers to change and creating buy-in and momentum. During the assess, plan, and early apply phases, communication themes include

▲ Strategic alignment
▲ Financial and operational advantages of deploying performance improvement
▲ How performance-improvement tools and methods will enhance and augment existing quality management processes and practices
▲ Goals for the deployment
▲ The roles of the people involved

Success stories from all industries should be communicated, always recognizing the unique culture of the healthcare organization. As practitioners are trained and projects and events are chartered and completed in the apply phase and onward, it is imperative that results are communicated and celebrated. Both the operational and financial impacts of the deployment should be communicated in the way and via the means and methods most meaningful to the target audience. Again, the target audience will determine the specifics.

When

The *when* of communication is determined by the target audience and a balance of influence and urgency. If key stakeholders will be involved later in the deployment and their influence is low to moderate, those communication activities can occur later in the apply phase. If the stakeholders' potential to affect the deployment is considerable and they will be involved in the early phases, it is critical to engage and inform them as early as possible. If the stakeholders' degree of influence and ability to affect the deployment are significant, then the communication plan should include a strategy and tactics to engage them even if they will not be actively involved until later in the deployment.

Where

The appropriate venue—*where* information is disseminated—generally is the one in which the target audience is accustomed to receiving important information. An initial announcement by leadership launching the deployment and communicating leadership vision, rationale, objectives, and expectations may be delivered in a special event. Many organizations hold what are commonly referred to as *town hall meetings*. These tend to be organization-wide events to emphasize that the performance-improvement deployment is not "business as usual" or the "flavor of the day." Subsequent messaging should be delivered in the venue most conducive to the free exchange of information. Those responsible for delivering the message therefore must be provided with adequate training and reference materials to address questions and concerns. Brevity and relevance are critical.

Why

One of the objectives of a communication plan is to generate a sense of urgency across all stakeholder groups. A key message must be delivered to each group that answers the question: *What's in it for me?* The reasons why a performance-improvement program is being deployed must be communicated in such a way that the rationale is obvious from each stakeholder's perspective. Just as the messages to the physicians and nurses must be customized to address their unique interests and concerns, the perspectives of each department and level of the organization also must be considered. For example, the marketing department would be most interested in performance improvement as a competitive advantage. Communicating quality initiatives as a differentiator has become more common in healthcare owing to the competition for recognition, such as the Malcolm Baldrige National Quality Award (Baldrige by Sector: Health Care 2010) and the American Nurses Credentialing Center Magnet status (ANCC Magnet Recognition Program 2010). However, it is just as important for the staff in dietary and sterile supply to understand how a performance-improvement program will affect the work they do each day and the value they deliver to their customers.

How

John Kotter assessed the reasons that transformation efforts fail and described the communication strategy necessary to avoid failure to sustain significant change. With regard to the *how* of communication, he describes a guiding principle: "Use every existing communication channel and opportunity." Successful communication plans use all the vehicles and media available. The best communication plans go beyond what currently exists and create innovative means and tools to generate interest in and enthusiasm and support for the performance-improvement deployment. Visual or graphic images capture the attention of busy professionals and communicate a maximum amount of information in a minimum amount of time. Making communication fun by using catchy phrases and games can be especially useful in the plan and early apply phases and later, when a plateau or a loss of momentum is likely to occur. In the latter, storyboards and testimonials of team members, champions, and customers celebrating the success of performance-improvement projects and events keep the message fresh and relevant. Examples of teaser posters are given in Figures 5.6 and 5.7.

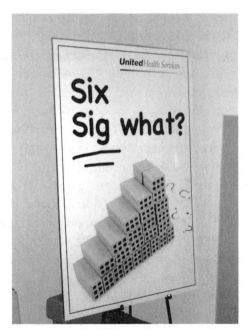

Figures 5.6 Teaser poster example.

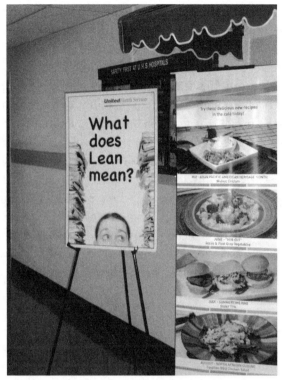

Figures 5.7   Another teaser poster example.

Communications Planning Summary

Examples of common and successful communication strategies during the launch of a performance-improvement program include presidential addresses to the staff at large, scripted presentations delivered by department managers to their staff, and presentations by committee heads at meetings or off-site retreats. More creative and less common examples include scavenger hunts and games using clues to lead workers step by step to the information being communicated. Songs and slogans have been used to pique interest in performance improvement and to cause people to ask questions in the early phases of a deployment, sparking interest and generating momentum. Means of ongoing communication include paper media such as newsletters, table tents in the cafeteria, posters, placards, and billboards. A host of electronic media options, such as television and videos,

Internet and intranet sites, and social media, can be useful. The best choice is determined by the audience being targeted. With the broad demographic and professional mix characteristic of a healthcare organization, Kotter's advice encourages a comprehensive and creative plan.

Accountability must be clearly established for each communication plan activity. The plan for *how* information about the deployment will be communicated must identify *to whom* the accountability for each action item belongs. This point person or persons provide regular, frequent status updates to the deployment team. At any given time, the deployment team needs to be aware of the current status of the communication plan so that adjustments or corrective actions can be taken when necessary. Communications management requires measures of progress toward objectives and *how well* the plan is working. These metrics should be defined and developed using the same principles as for any other performance indicator. A well-executed communication plan is a strong predictor of a successful performance-improvement deployment.

Project Selection

"You can't move so fast that you try to change the mores faster than people can accept it. That doesn't mean you do nothing, but it means that you do the things that need to be done according to priority."
—ELEANOR ROOSEVELT, FORMER FIRST LADY OF THE UNITED STATES

Project selection is the most critical and most challenging activity in launching performance-improvement deployment—the Achilles' heel of these initiatives and critical to any short- or long-term business-change program. Selecting the right projects and events ranks second only to leadership support as the factor most closely linked to performance-improvement deployment success—and failure. Performance-improvement projects and events represent a significant investment of time and other resources, not the least of which is strategic focus. Deploying resources as valuable as performance-improvement practitioners to fix the *wrong* problems is the worst kind of waste, an observation that is sure to be made by those monitoring the return on investment for a performance-improvement program. One of the reasons that training practitioners and sending them forth *to fix* things consistently fails as a deployment strategy is that the projects and events these newly trained practitioners select or are assigned are almost certain to be the wrong ones. As a result, projects and events never reach fruition, fail to meet milestones or to produce the anticipated return on investment, or are abandoned altogether as leadership focus wanes or shifts elsewhere.

What is the *right* project or event? The answer to this question depends on the maturity of the deployment, the expertise and availability of practitioners, and shifting environmental and organizational conditions. Projects and events must be clearly linked to organizational strategy. The process for selecting performance-improvement projects and events should be part of the cycle of strategic planning, performance measurement, and financial planning and budgeting. Only performance-improvement opportunities, problems, or performance gaps determined to be of strategic importance should become chartered projects and events. Once identified, the right project or event must be scoped appropriately. Too narrow and the results will not make an appreciable impact on organizational objectives. Too broad and the project or event will take too long or never reach closure, consuming valuable resources and leadership patience. "Boil the ocean" or "Solve world hunger" projects ultimately will fail or have to be redefined. Finally, the right projects and events meet the criteria for project success. This does not mean that *difficult* projects should not be chartered, but rather that the factors linked to success should be considered as part of the decision-making process.

Opportunities being considered should meet certain criteria. While each organization needs to determine its own criteria, some possible considerations include

▲ Does it affect the system constraint?
▲ Is the project linked directly to strategic goals?
▲ Does the process relate to key business objectives?
▲ Will project success improve customer satisfaction?
▲ Does the process occur frequently?
▲ Does a performance gap exist?
▲ Is process ownership clearly established?
▲ Is the scope of the project appropriate?
▲ Can the project be completed in six months or less?

▲ Are the needed resources (i.e., people, time, capital and data) available?
▲ Is the project independent of other improvement initiatives (including automation)?

Project Sources

Selecting the right projects or events at the right time and for the right practitioners at the right point in their development is somewhat subjective. It requires leadership commitment and active involvement, as well as the guidance of an advanced performance-improvement practitioner. It is a process that can be understood, measured, and managed. A successful deployment and effective, productive practitioners depend on doing project and event selection right.

Identification of performance-improvement projects and events is an unavoidable responsibility of leadership that cannot be delegated. As discussed earlier, opportunity identification is a critical outcome from the JumpStart and planning activities conducted early in a performance-improvement deployment. Some sources that are available include

▲ Patient satisfaction surveys
▲ Hospital survey on patient safety culture
▲ Joint Commission periodic performance review
▲ Center for Medicare and Medicaid Services (CMS) core measures
▲ Healthcare Effectiveness Data and Information Set (HEDIS)
▲ National Database of Nursing Quality Indicators
▲ Internal metrics

Projects are also identified through evaluation of core business processes and any gaps in performance that are present. Once core processes have been identified and mapped to a level where metrics and data exist, each process is assessed in terms of cost, quality, and time. Further assessment frequently requires additional information or subject matter expertise.

Constraints

In the integrated approach to performance improvement, identification of system constraints is an important source of project opportunities.

Identification of system constraints that present performance-improvement opportunities and possible projects and events begins with the creation of an Intermediate Objectives (IO) map and focused current reality tree (fCRT), tools that were described in the thinking processes section of Chapter 2. The IO map identifies critical success factors (CSFs) necessary to achieve strategic goals. If the CSFs are not attained, then undesirable effects (UDEs) are identified. Each UDE then is evaluated for cause. Core drivers—factors or areas connecting multiple UDEs—are determined, as H. William Dettmer originally advised in the book, *Goldratt's Theory of Constraints: A Systems Approach to Continuous Improvement.* An fCRT is used to identify which core drivers, if positively affected, will have a profound and immediate impact on the organization's ability to achieve strategic objectives.

Strategic Imperatives Identified by Leadership

A final source of potential projects that cannot be discounted are the *strategic imperatives* identified by leadership. Strategic imperatives identified by leadership are added to the opportunity portfolio. Caution must be exercised when translating opportunities, regardless of their source, to potential performance-improvement projects and events. Management hot buttons or pet projects do not necessarily make the best performance-improvement projects or events. They must be subjected to the same prioritization and selection criteria as those obtained from any other source. It is not uncommon for a leader to endeavor to address an agenda under the guise of a performance-improvement opportunity.

Project Prioritization

Once identified, opportunities must be evaluated and prioritized. These prioritized opportunities should be documented in a standard, easily assessable format. The format of a project portfolio, also called a *project hopper* or *opportunity database*, may be as simple as an Excel workbook or as complex as an intranet or software application specifically designed for the purpose. The portfolio must be viewed as a *living document* used to store a comprehensive and ongoing list of performance-improvement opportunities that may or may not become chartered or completed projects and events. Appropriate use of the portfolio ensures that the right project or event is chartered at the right time and when the right methodology and right practitioner are available.

The structure, process, responsibility, and nomenclature for adding opportunities to the portfolio, as well as the process for identifying, selecting, prioritizing, and chartering projects, are critical elements of deployment infrastructure that must be developed during the plan phase. This is the primary operational responsibility of the deployment team, once leadership strategy and prioritization criteria have been determined. The objective is not the quantity of opportunities identified but rather that every important opportunity is considered. It is not unusual for a seemingly unwieldy number of opportunities, as many as 100 or more, to be identified during a JumpStart and remain that high moving forward—some being worked, others added.

The structure and elements of a project and event portfolio can be as unique as the healthcare organization it is intended to serve. However, there are several standard elements. The project portfolio must include some unique, usually alphanumeric identifier so that each entry can be linked to the files, documents, and data associated with it. This essential infrastructural element ensures that there is clarity of definition, lack of unintentional overlap, and no duplication of effort. The ability to reference portfolio entries is important when replication of projects and events begins to occur as the deployment matures, generally in the apply phase. A brief description of the opportunity and identity of a process owner and a champion should be included. Some estimate of the likely methodology that is based on a preliminary understanding of the problem is important for the allocation of resources, including time. The most important elements of the portfolio are the following:

▲ Core drivers
▲ Links to strategic goals
▲ Prioritization criteria

Factors established by the leadership team during the plan phase will guide initial prioritization of project opportunities. The relationship between the opportunity and each strategic goal, usually qualitative (such as low, medium, high or a simple yes or no), prioritization criteria and weights developed by the leadership and deployment teams, and core drivers (yes or no) are used to determine whether a project or event will be considered an immediate priority for performance-improvement intervention. There are many sophisticated tools and methods that can be used to prioritize performance-improvement projects and events. The best tool is one that considers all the essential dimensions, makes a clear distinction between rankings (first, second, third, and so on), and provides an ongoing means of collecting performance-improvement opportunities and linking them to projects and events, as well as any related documentation or information associated with them.

The objective of these methods is a rank-ordered list of strategically aligned projects prioritized according to criteria defined and weighted by leadership. Ultimately, each of these methods relies on human intelligence and judgment, some qualitative evaluation of the strength of a relationship, to assign a quantitative ranking. What is important is that the criteria selected by leadership reflect the strategic intent and imperatives of the organization and that they are clearly defined.

If a criteria-based approach is used, each criterion should be weighted to reflect its relative strategic importance, and the weight assigned must allow for adequate differentiation. If every criterion is weighted the same, it is difficult, if not impossible, to distinguish between an important project or event that *should be chartered sometime* and a critical project or event that *must be chartered now*. Conversely, weighting one criterion so heavily that a certain type of project is unlikely to ever be chartered can skew the selection process. A leadership team may emphasize *financial return* so heavily that only projects with a strong financial return are likely to be chartered. Conversely, they may place the overriding emphasis on *quality of care* such that only opportunities with the potential to affect patient safety or satisfaction will be chartered. As stated frequently throughout this book, a dual focus is necessary to operate as a viable business. Other common selection criteria include

▲ Customer/patient impact
▲ Opportunity for replication
▲ Risk
▲ Availability of special skills or tools
▲ Process cycle frequency
▲ Return on investment

There has been considerable effort invested in developing more *quantitative* methods of distinguishing an immediate priority from a project or event of lesser urgency. Some take a practical approach of combining filtering and prioritization. Others take a very systematic approach. The *structure-conduct-performance (S-C-P) approach* incorporates strength, weakness, opportunity, and threats (SWOT) and valuable, rare, imitable, and organized (VRIO) analyses into a project-selection algorithm such as the one proposed by Mark R. Tellier in his article, "DMAIC Project Selection Using a Systematic Approach." Others, while structured, are less complex— such as the simple point-allocation system Drew Peregrim suggests in his article, "Use Point System for Better Six Sigma Project Selection." In the book *Lean Six Sigma*, Michael George suggests that the ultimate success of a performance-improvement program depends on an inclusive approach to project identification using both top-down and bottom-up opportunity-identification strategies. Top-down strategies include

▲ Balanced scorecard
▲ Strategic gap analysis
▲ Financial analyses, such as the value driver
▲ Customer requirements derived from Kano analyses
▲ Process classification methods such as the process edge approach

Bottom-up strategies include

▲ Brainstorming
▲ Affinitizing
▲ Screening ideas solicited from all levels of the organization

In the journal *Business Process Management*, Kumar, Antony, and Cho present a complex hybrid method using an analytical hierarchy process and a project desirability matrix. The *analytical hierarchy process* is designed to determine the relative priorities or weights to be assigned to different criteria and alternatives, whereas the *project desirability matrix* compares effort required and impact of the project.

Some annotation of the status of the opportunity is necessary, such as "chartered," "define phase," "scheduled," and/or "complete." Finally, some accommodation for notes regarding status is useful, such as "pending training" or "data collection to quantify problem statement." The owner of the portfolio, generally the deployment leader or his or her designee, should be able to use the tool to proficiently report the current status of performance-improvement opportunities, projects, and events to the executive steering committee at any time. In especially sophisticated models, the current status of the project or event is displayed on a color-coded scorecard or in dashboard format, some having the capability to drill down or link to files, documents, metrics, and data.

All these methods have their advantages and disadvantages. However, it can become confusing to a practitioner who is uncertain which criteria takes precedence. For clarity, if the system's constraint has been identified, as we highly recommend, then priority should be given to get the most out of the constraint and even break it if needed.

First Projects

The *improvement opportunity portfolio* is a living document that evolves as the deployment matures. Project and event selection processes and criteria change over time—from a pragmatic and tactical approach in the initial phases of a deployment to an increasingly strategic approach as the deployment matures. Initially, the sources of performance-improvement opportunities include system-based value-stream analysis (SystemVSA), system constraint analysis, and strategic gap analysis, as well as issues and gaps identified by leadership. The criteria for selecting initial projects and events will emphasize tangible, immediate results to create support and momentum. *Visibility* is sometimes added as a criterion for selecting inaugural projects and events. This sequence ensures that initial performance-improvement endeavors target well-known problems and generate as much excitement and momentum as possible to launch the deployment. The criteria for selection of a training project differ from those when experienced practitioners are available. Later on, practitioner effectiveness is an important deployment metric, and financial benefits and deployment return on investment increase in relative importance. This shift is reflected in revised criteria or weighting of criteria. The source of opportunities also changes as the deployment matures, from JumpStart events to the balanced scorecard, and as a natural outcome of the strategic planning cycle.

Critical Chain Project Management (CCPM) for Performance-Improvement Project Portfolios

As summarized in Chapter 2, critical chain project management principles are applicable to both individual process-improvement projects and the performance-improvement project portfolio. This is especially true for high-priority projects. Most green belts and some black belts work on performance-improvement projects on a part-time basis. As a result, depending on the priority set by the leadership, projects can be delayed significantly. Highlighting the impact of bad multitasking to project champions and process-improvement practitioners at a minimum is recommended first and foremost. As shown in Figure 5.8, project schedules with and without multitasking underline the delays expected when multitasking occurs.

There is a common misperception that refraining from multitasking means that people are solely and totally committed to the project and nothing else until the task is completed. This technique is sometimes not practical given the resources available. An adaptation of no multitasking can mean that, for a certain number of hours per day (normally not fewer than four hours), people are dedicated to the project and nothing else until each task at hand is completed. One thing to remember when employing critical chain project management is that the rule about no multitasking

Sample Timeline by Phase

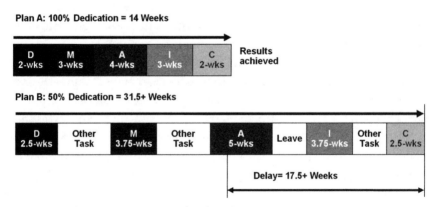

Figure 5.8   Impact of multitasking on project execution.

must be applied consistently for this concept to succeed fully. For critical projects, we recommend following project *run rules*, also known as *right of way*, to support people working on the project.

Conduct a daily 15-minute "stand up" meeting:

▲ Provide a time to preview what is coming that day. Questions to ask include, "How many days are remaining on the project? Will you make your commitments? Do you have any barriers to completing your tasks on time?"

▲ List actions on a flip chart for all to see, and leave it visible until the next meeting. Assign each action to someone on the team, and have a 24-hour resolution suspense.

Manage constraints:

▲ Assign team members to only one task at a time.

▲ Identify and manage (with the sponsor or executive leader) the constraints associated with the project, such as the availability of time, people, data, and stakeholder attention.

▲ Prioritize project tasks based on the charter and the project deliverables. For example, some data-collection tasks are more important to project success than others.

▲ Do not assign new tasks until previously assigned tasks are complete.

Use visual controls:

▲ Post the project schedule in a designated project area. Identify the people working on the project by name, and create a sign of some kind to indicate that they are on a critical performance-improvement project. For example, at a major organization, a special tape, like crime scene tape, is used to indicate that people are working on a Six Sigma project.

▲ Have project run rules to support people working on the project (known as *right of way*), and protect them from distractions.

Implement special team procedures:

▲ Designate one or two hours per day to work on a performance-improvement project team. Expect the team to work on nothing else during that period: No phone calls and no informal meetings are allowed. The project team is, in essence, "locked down."

▲ All phone calls received during this period are directed to voicemail. The recorded greeting indicates that the team member cannot come to the phone because he or she is working on a critical performance-improvement project. The greeting directs callers to contact an assistant for emergencies and states that other calls will be returned during office hours.

▲ Use a "war room" to display and preserve project work. This eliminates setup time and prevents loss of critical information.

These rules accelerate the completion of performance-improvement projects by using critical chain project management concepts. For the most vital projects, a full critical chain project management implementation should be considered.

Conclusion

This chapter covered the transition from identifying performance gaps and improvement opportunities to the development of an action plan for addressing them. The plan should contain the necessary details to ensure timely and consistent execution as well as be robust enough to adapt to an ever-changing environment. It should address the ubiquitous who, when, what, where, and how.

After the assess and plan phases, it is time to *apply*. Next, Chapter 6 covers applying performance-improvement tools in healthcare organizations from chartering projects and events to the constitution of those elements themselves.

Application of the Right Tool to the Right Problem

"Knowing is not enough; we must apply. Willing is not enough; we must do."

—JOHANN WOLFGANG VON GOETHE,
MASTER OF MODERN GERMAN LITERATURE

This chapter focuses on the application of appropriate performance-improvement tools to achieve the desired results. Depending on the nature of the improvement opportunities, specific toolsets and methodologies are used. These include quick hits, rapid improvement workshops, Six Sigma projects, and Constraints Management solutions.

Project Chartering and Execution

Opportunities for performance improvement present themselves in many ways. In the assess phase, numerous improvement opportunities should have been identified and documented. As a result of the investigation into the identified gaps, improvement actions will be initiated. There are numerous approaches to performance improvement. The following will be addressed:

▲ Quick hit improvements
▲ Process-based value-stream analysis (ProcessVSA)
▲ Rapid improvement workshops
▲ Six Sigma projects
▲ Constraints Management applications
▲ Executive actions
▲ Critical chain project management (CCPM)

Project Chartering

All improvement efforts should be viewed as a project. In *Juran's Quality Control Handbook*, Joseph M. Juran contends that all improvement happens project by project and in no other way. When improvement efforts are viewed as projects, then basic principles of project management should apply. Each project should have a charter. Without a written charter, team members cannot be sure that they understand the sponsor's expectations and are in proper alignment with organizational needs.

In an early article on the use of charters in quality improvement in healthcare, Nancy Wilkinson and John Moran defined a *charter* as a document developed by the sponsor that empowers the team to act. The team charter sets the foundation and direction for the project and the team.

In the article, "Six Sigma and Beyond," Thomas Pyzdek maintains that the project definition is made explicit in the project charter. He further reinforces that the project sponsor is responsible for developing the charter and that it then provides the practitioners with the authority to apply organizational resources to project activities.

Charters are useful to the team and contribute to the overall efficacy of the performance-improvement effort in several ways. Charters are often used as a facilitation tool. Viewing the life cycle of a project in human terms, Richard Roble cites specific uses of the charter during adolescence as a focal point to keep the team on track, as well as during adulthood to monitor performance against objectives. If a charter is not given proper attention, the chips are stacked against a successful performance-improvement event from the outset.

It is the responsibility of leaders at all levels of an organization to serve as champions. Within their respective area of operational control, they are directly responsible for the outcome of a business unit's performance-improvement efforts. In this role, they sponsor improvement activities and develop project charters in coordination with the project selection and prioritization process. These efforts should be aligned with the overall business strategy. Champions should actively influence, motivate, and drive performance-improvement efforts.

Sponsoring Projects

When sponsoring projects, champions should manage the scope of the project and ensure that sufficient resources are available. For champions, the advantages of familiarity with the benefit validation process and skillful coordination with stakeholders should not be underestimated. Champions take actions necessary to overcome roadblocks to project success and provide feedback and approvals during project tollgates or briefings. Working closely with the program management office, champions communicate their performance-improvement efforts to the executive leadership team.

The level at which performance-improvement tools are applied affects the approval process. When appropriate improvement resources are within the control of the owner of a given process, that owner normally can initiate efforts without prior approval or coordination. When performance-improvement resources are controlled centrally, requirements for their use must be reviewed and prioritized against other organizational requirements. Under either paradigm, quick hits are, by definition, within the control of the process owner and require no approval.

Improvement Approach Selection

There is more than one way to approach a problem. It is important that each case be examined critically to determine the most appropriate approach. It is not until the problem is reviewed and a basic understanding of the process is gained that the best approach can be determined. Figure 6.1 shows an improvement methodology selection tree. Prioritized problems can come from JumpStart sessions, which include system-based value-stream analysis (SystemVSA), system constraints analysis, and strategic gap analysis as critical components. A project is selected from the project selection prioritization matrix, as explained in Chapter 5. Performance-improvement projects also can come from ProcessVSAs, which include the five focusing steps in an analysis of the current state and the design of the future state. The improvement approach selection tree can be used to help determine the best performance-improvement tool for the issue at hand.

When the root cause is known, a rapid improvement workshop should be considered. When both the root cause and the solution to a problem are known, an intuitive option would be to take direct action to mitigate the issue—a quick hit or a Constraints Management solution that addresses that specific problem. For example, if the problem is that information technology (IT) projects are taking too long, then a critical chain project

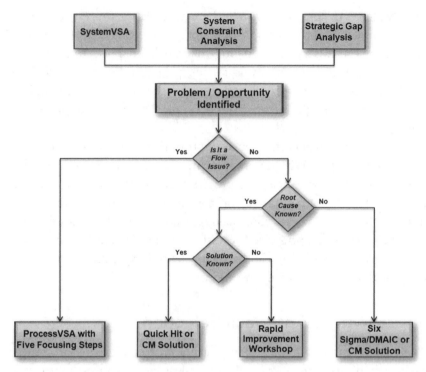

Figure 6.1 Improvement methodology selection tree.

management solution would be appropriate to consider. If the root cause is known but the solution is not, then a rapid improvement workshop or, again, a Constraints Management solution would be appropriate depending on the nature of the root cause. The Constraints Management thinking processes tool is an effective alternative to determining the root cause of a healthcare organization's problems. As described below, its roadmap is suitable for a rapid improvement workshop as well.

When confronted with a problem and the root cause is not known, additional data and analysis are required to determine the root cause. For such instances a Six Sigma project would be appropriate, depending on the context. The thinking processes of Constraints Management can be used during DMAIC phases for root-cause analysis as well as solution development. Some organizations can gain sufficient understanding without detailed data analysis by using logical thinking embedded in thinking processes leading to faster problem solution.

In his Theory of Constraints International Certification Organization (TOCICO) 2004 Conference presentation, "Integrating the TOC Thinking Process and Six Sigma," Chris Zephro detailed his use of the thinking processes at Seagate, the world's largest hard-drive manufacturer. Specifically, use of the current reality tree (CRT) in the analyze phase and use of the future reality tree (FRT) and the conflict cloud (CC) in the improve phase are recommended. Zephro found that use of these tools increased the quality of project results dramatically. Projects became more focused. The thinking processes also provided more clearly defined solution paths, and they reduced resistance to buy-in for proposed solutions. When these tools were applied at Seagate, Zephro calculated that the project completion rate increased by 80 percent, and the number of projects completed within 3 months increased by 70 percent. Graduating "transactional belts" voted CRT, FRT, and CC as the most useful Six Sigma tools in every wave since their introduction. Zephro also added that the CRT has become the primary tool used for project mining.

Implementation of critical chain project management (CCPM) for performance-improvement projects is strongly recommended, where applicable. When a problem is related to project delays, which is quite common for IT applications, the CCPM solution of Constraints Management can be a viable option. Improvement teams still need to analyze the root causes of project delays because there may be additional root causes besides multitasking, student syndrome, and work expansion according to time allocated (Parkinson's law)—common root causes that CCPM addresses effectively. In many cases, IT applications are subcontracted, and hospital IT resources are not sufficient to meet the demand for new or modified functions and interface requirements. Chapter 2 details how IT departments (and a few other departments) are permanent bottlenecks of hospitals and that they should be managed as such using the five focusing steps.

If the purpose of the project is to deal with problems related to very high stock levels or stock-outs of medications and supplies, the replenishment approach of Constraints Management could provide a powerful solution if the hospital can establish the infrastructure required for its application and manage change effectively, which entails a major paradigm shift, as detailed in Chapter 2.

If waiting times are unacceptably long with a lot of variation, the logistics solutions of Constraints Management should be considered, especially in emergency departments. Strategic decisions need to be made as to whether physicians or number of beds will be treated as the system constraints. In addition, tracking of patient treatment status, almost always with IT applications, would be needed, as described in Chapter 2. Logistical and replenishment solutions employ buffer management to absorb variation. Critical chain requires use of project buffers in a very dynamic manner.

Constraints Management applications, as well as other adaptable preexisting solutions, should be kept in mind during improvement projects so as to avoid "reinventing the wheel." We do not rederive the chemical formula for aspirin every time it is dispensed. Let there be no confusion: We do not condone one-sized-fits-all solutions nor boxed products to resolve problems where the root cause is unknown without applying the thinking processes, a Six Sigma project, or at least a standalone root-cause analysis tool. However, included within the recommended toolsets of Lean, Six Sigma, Constraints Management, and even the theory of inventive problem solving (TRIZ), which will be described near the end of this chapter, are broad guidelines for applying tested principles to adapting unique solutions tailored to the specific characteristics of a given environment. We do *not* advocate simply aping another organization's best practices and calling it "benchmarking" absent understanding. While doing so may expedite a solution, the performance-improvement team runs a very real risk that it may be missing *the* critical factor at the bottom of the healthcare organization's specific issue, and problems will fester beyond the project's slated completion date.

Process-Level Value Stream Analysis

A process-level VSA (ProcessVSA) is an approach to analyzing a process to identify and eliminate non-value-adding activities as well as to develop procedures to manage bottlenecks effectively and break those bottlenecks when needed. It is also a planning tool that uses process mapping to help understand how material and information flow through a process, as well as to identify constraints at the process level. Additionally, ideal and future state process maps are developed that focus future improvement activities within that process. ProcessVSAs are conducted by following a product's or service's path from suppliers to customers. Once the current state of the process is mapped, it is then analyzed to identify waste, inefficiencies, constraints, and other improvement opportunities. After areas of opportunity have been identified, an ideal state map is created to serve as a benchmark. Then a future state map is created showing how the material and information should flow and how the process bottleneck should be managed, if there is one. Champions are designated to sponsor improvement efforts by first determining the best approach. Finally, an action plan is prepared to move from the current state to the future state of the process. This action plan should include recommendations for future rapid improvement events, quick hits, and DMAIC and Constraints Management projects.

A ProcessVSA generally is run as a single event lasting five days or less. There are three phases to this process: pre-event, event, and post-event. Each phase has a series of sequential steps to complete for a successful outcome. Figure 6.2 shows the ProcessVSA pre-event roadmap.

Pre-event

Selecting the ProcessVSA Champion

Because healthcare organizations tend to be separated into functions and departments, very often it is difficult to find a single manager who owns the entire process proposed for analysis. While the champion may or may not be the process owner, in this key role, he or she is directly responsible for the outcome of the ProcessVSA. This critical role is often assigned to a senior manager because processes usually cross managerial boundaries within organizations. In addition to monitoring the team's progress and providing strategic direction to ensure alignment with organizational goals,

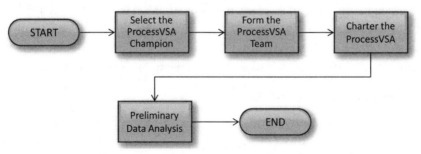

Figure 6.2 ProcessVSA pre-event roadmap.

the champion also removes barriers to team success. The champion should have sufficient authority to assign resources and ensure implementation of the resulting process improvements. Champions are selected similarly in rapid improvement workshops and Six Sigma projects.

Forming the ProcessVSA Team

Selection of team members is as important as selecting the champion because of the experience and process knowledge they bring to the ProcessVSA. A well-rounded ProcessVSA team includes people with deep subject matter expertise, those who work in the process with customers. IT technical experts should be on the team to answer automation or system capability questions, and as appropriate, so should customers and suppliers to the process as well. Teams often benefit from having a financial subject matter expert—if not on the team proper, then on call as needed to ensure that costs can be captured accurately.

Team members should be enthusiastic about the potential for improvement and willing to look outside the box for solutions. Of course, team members also must have the time to participate in the ProcessVSA. One of the challenges for the champion and performance-improvement deployment as a whole is that it is desirable to have an organization's best people participate, yet the best people quite often have other responsibilities they must perform as part of their daily duties that leave them with very little time to work on other tasks. Assigning adequate resources to ProcessVSA and other performance-improvement opportunities is one of the greatest challenges for the champion and advocates of continuous improvement. Companies committed to continuous performance improvement will find ways to ensure that teams have the right mix of skills.

ProcessVSA teams are relatively small, with enough people to share the work equitably, but not so many members that the team is unmanageable. Core teams usually are comprised of about four to seven people; other subject matter experts can participate on an on-call basis. Teams are formed similarly in rapid improvement workshops and Six Sigma projects.

Chartering the ProcessVSA

The charter is the covenant between the team and the organization to deliver on the promise of rational performance improvement. At a minimum, the charter spells out the mission or purpose of the ProcessVSA, whether it is being launched in response to customer service concerns or to the organization's strategic goals. The purpose is the business case, the rationale for committing resources to the ProcessVSA; it defines the value of the effort. A blank charter is shown in the Appendix.

Charters also identify deliverables, the ProcessVSA schedule or timeline, team members, champion, the lead practitioner, process boundaries, alignment with strategic intent, and metrics. Deliverables, which also may be specified as objectives in the charter, identify the results the team will deliver. The ProcessVSA boundaries, or scope, identify the beginning and end of the process to be analyzed. Just as high-level process maps help to define scope, ProcessVSA boundaries clearly identify the process—or portions of very large or complex processes—to be studied by the team.

The ProcessVSA charter should indicate whether the targeted process aligns with overarching corporate goals or with another business imperative, such as a process performance problem that affects regulatory compliance. Likewise, the metrics identified in the charter should reflect strategic intent. While the analyses result in improved flow time and reduced waste, which can be measured in dollars, there may be other measures that should be tracked as part of the ProcessVSA, such as patient satisfaction, employee satisfaction, and reductions in errors and defects. Rapid improvement workshops and Six Sigma projects are chartered similarly to ProcessVSAs.

Preliminary Data Analysis

Prior to the event, the lead practitioner should collect and review all available process information. This should include, but not be limited to, existing process documentation (i.e., standard operating procedures, process maps, and previous improvement activities) and any available data. Available data may include process cycle times, customer wait times, defect rates, and any other information that may assist the team in improving the process flow. Figure 6.3 shows the ProcessVSA event roadmap. In rapid

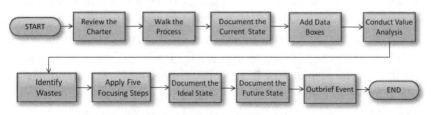

Figure 6.3 ProcessVSA event roadmap.

improvement workshops and Six Sigma projects, preliminary data are analyzed similarly.

Event

Reviewing the Charter

The event charter is the primary document to guide the progress of the event. All team members must fully understand the components. Review the charter for the following elements with the team:

- ▲ Purpose
- ▲ Alignment with strategic intent
- ▲ Business case
- ▲ Deliverables
- ▲ Schedule
- ▲ Boundaries of the process
- ▲ Team members

Walking the Process

While the ProcessVSA lead practitioner may assign specific tasks to individual team members later, early in the ProcessVSA, the team literally should be *walking the process* in order to observe the work firsthand. Walking the process entails following the entire workflow from start to finish, taking on the perspective of the unit or patient where it makes sense, in addition to any work done behind the scenes as part of the process under investigation. This is important because how work actually gets done is quite often nothing like the way it is described in procedures, so the team needs to see for itself how materials and information flow through the process.

Documenting Current-State Flow

During the process walk, the team should be collecting data on material and information flow not only in terms of what types of materials, items, and information flow through the process but also in terms of how. It should be noted that the ProcessVSA does not use the traditional value-stream map. The map of the *current state* is a detailed process-level map accomplished with a degree of detail that allows for identification of value-added/non-value-added activities and other forms of waste as well as constraints.

The most important thing to remember about process mapping is that the map is a visual representation of the process, so it is essential that the process map be comprehensible. Using advanced mapping icons can add clutter and confusion—if they are not necessary to *tell the story* of the process, don't use them.

Once the team has completed mapping the process, it should have a map that illustrates the work process, as well as data about overall flow time, wait time, process time, rework, bottlenecks, and other information necessary for analysis. Two other graphic displays that are useful are the spaghetti and circle diagrams. *Spaghetti diagrams* show how people and materials move in physical space: Do people have to walk away from one station to another? Do people cross paths? Spaghetti diagrams help to illustrate distance, which the team also collects while walking the process. While the spaghetti diagram, as shown in Figure 6.4, is a powerful tool for processes involving physical movement, the *circle diagram*, which is used normally to show handoffs in the process, also can be used to show the flow of data or information.

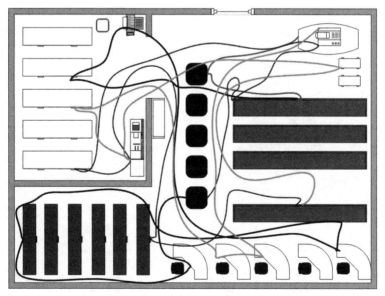

Figure 6.4 Spaghetti diagram.

Conducting Value Analysis

A good current-state map will show where decisions or inspections occur in the process, such as in Figure 6.5. Decisions or inspections, which are represented by diamonds on the map, can be good indicators of where waste or inefficiency hides in the process because there are two opportunities for errors to occur:

▲ An item or information is *passed* when it should have failed.
▲ An item or information is *failed* when it should have passed.

When the team is satisfied that it has all the data on the current state that it can reasonably collect, it looks at the detailed steps in the process to determine where there is waste or inefficiency. This step is sometimes called *assigning value classes* because the team decides whether each step adds value (*value-added*), does not add value (*non-value-added*), or is required by regulation or other mandate (*non-value-added but necessary* or *business-value-added*). These are normally documented using green, red, and yellow to designate value-added, non-value-added, and non-value-added but

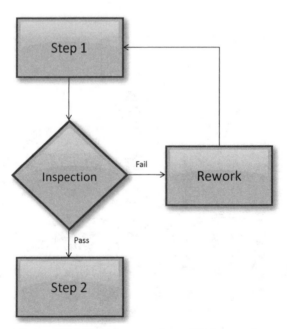

Figure 6.5 Inspection—value-added example.

necessary/business-value-added, respectively. Note that space on the data box is allocated for the placement of commercially available colored dot stickers. The team should be ruthless in assigning value classifications to the current-state map; that is, the non-value-added but necessary category ought to be used only when there is a law, regulation, or mandate that can be identified specifically requiring the activity. In general, any kind of inspection—whether it is a review of a document or obtaining an additional signature—is considered non-value-added, and the current-state map should be coded accordingly. ProcessVSA teams will find initially that very few steps in a process are truly value-added, so it is normal to find current-state maps with lots of red and yellow coding.

Identifying Other Waste and Constraints

In addition to designating certain activities as value added or not, the team will identify other barriers to process flow or efficiency. In most instances, these can be easily related to one of the seven common categories of waste. Figure 1.5 (in Chapter 1) shows the typical types of waste. These are equally applicable in both manufacturing and transactional processes.

In addition to these common wastes, all processes have a system constraint. If that constraint is a resource that cannot handle the demand placed on it, then there is a key bottleneck inhibiting the capacity of the process. Bottlenecks are not always obvious. When walking the process, the discovery and identification of work in process (WIP) are excellent indications of process flow issues. WIP takes many forms, from specimens awaiting lab tests to customers queuing for service. Once a process constraint is identified, the team needs to ensure that the constraint is clearly annotated in the current-state map. It also should be clearly noted in the project identification worksheet. Initial efforts to improve Throughput should be focused on the constraint of the whole system.

Applying the Five Focusing Steps

As described in Chapters 1 and 2, the five focusing steps of Constraint Management provide an excellent means to mitigate a constraint. During a ProcessVSA, at a bare minimum, it is appropriate to perform step one, *identify* the constraint. The team should strive for agreement on the constraint identified, but facilitation is recommended to ensure that disagreement does not become a hindrance to team unity or progression through the five focusing steps. If consensus cannot be reached, hopefully enough of a dialog will have occurred between the disagreeing parties that those holding the less popular position are at least persuaded that the other side's case has some merit. Even if it is not their preferred option, all members of the team should be convinced that improving the constraint identified at least in some way could benefit the process.

In the next step of a ProcessVSA, the team will be called on to design ideal and future states of the process. In so doing, it also should be performing steps two and three, *exploiting* the constraint to get the most out of it and *subordinating* other resources and steps in the process to the decision to support the constraint. Redesigning steps in the processes, reallocating work among resources, and rewriting standard operating procedures are just a few examples of where steps two and three could be applied within the scope of a ProcessVSA.

Depending on whether the team feels that sufficient gains can be achieved through steps two and three, it also may be appropriate to explore use of step four—*elevate* the constraint. Elevating a bad policy constraint can necessitate amending it or even breaking the policy altogether. If the constraint is a resource, step four finds some means to increase capacity, such as bringing old equipment back online during periods of peak demand or reassigning staff members who are working on nonbottlenecks to work on bottlenecks. Especially if it will not be broken, the team needs to focus on how to get the most out of the bottleneck.

If the team makes the decision to break a constraint, it should plan not only how it will be broken but also where it will move subsequently. Given the strategic nature of the location of the constraint, the more drastically a constraint is being altered, the closer the team should be in consultation with the champion. Since elevating the constraint often requires investment in new resources, a recommendation that the executive leadership team consider doing so may be well suited for inclusion in a plan of action and milestones. Opportunities to exploit and subordinate the constraint that could not be accomplished within the ProcessVSA event's time span also are listed. The plan of action and milestones will be defined in its own section below.

While the spirit of the five focusing steps should be imbued throughout the ProcessVSA, we recommend that time be allocated in every ProcessVSA

CASE STUDY

A Process-Level Value-Stream Analysis with Five Focusing Steps

At a hospital system, the cycle times for interventional radiology (IR) and CT scan (CT) procedures were too long, compromising patient Throughput, creating backlogs, and limiting capacity in IR and CT and on outpatient-care units. A ProcessVSA was conducted with a goal to improve procedure cycle time and patient Throughput, thereby increasing IR and CT capacity. By including the five focusing steps of Constraints Management in this activity as an integral part of the analysis, the team was able to reveal not only non-value-added activities, but also constraints that limit Throughput. In step one, two critical resource constraints were immediately obvious as the main process constraint candidates: the interventional radiologists and the procedure suites within which IR procedures were performed.

A major policy constraint was scheduling and placement of IR patients. Procedures were scheduled in calendar two-hour blocks of time without consideration of the anticipated cycle time for the procedure ordered or the patient's medical needs. Patients were assigned beds on hospital units without regard to complexity, prerequisite laboratory determinations or preparations, anticipated recovery needs, expected cycle time of the procedure, or proximity to the procedure suite. All IR and CT patients were scheduled and managed in the same manner regardless of procedure or medical condition. This homogenization created inefficiencies and redundancies, overutilization of radiology resources, increased IR cycle times, and decreased Throughput that contributed to procedure backlogs.

Artificial constraints included use of radiology nurses for nonnursing tasks that could be handled by less expensive staff. These nonnursing tasks included answering the telephone, coordinating transportation of outpatients to and from IR, communicating delays up and down the value stream, and untangling scheduling problems when procedures were added to the schedule. Root causes for delays and backlogs were identified, and a plan of action and milestones was developed.

CASE STUDY

The high degree of variability in procedure cycle time was attributed to patients arriving for procedures without the necessary prerequisite laboratory determinations, preparations, or documents. Because there was no patient care and preparation area in the IR department (another resource constraint), the patient occupied the procedure suite while documents and consents were obtained, laboratory samples were drawn and results reviewed, and other preparations were completed, if necessary. This created rework, compounded delays, and constrained flow. If the IR staff was not able to obtain the required documentation or laboratory results were not sufficient to proceed, then the procedure would be rescheduled. This lack of preparedness was identified as a primary cause of compounding delays and wasting IR capacity.

A separate rapid improvement workshop was chartered to develop a set of protocols to guide and standardize scheduling, staffing, level of care, bed assignment, completion of prerequisites for procedures, and preparation for and recovery after procedures. As the team brainstormed what is critical to quality, team members struggled to *keep it simple* and yet create a tool that was comprehensive enough to meet all the needs identified.

One of the interventional radiologists on the team compared the functionality needed to tollgates on a nearby bridge: Some patients have a speed pass; some need exact change. The key is getting every patient into the lane that best meets his or her needs. This analogy sparked the team's creativity, and it quickly became obvious that an algorithm was the better solution.

Three IR pathways were identified by the improvement team to get the most out of the system's constraints (step two)—removing all non-value-added activity from the procedure suites and eliminating waiting and transportation for the radiologists. These pathways guide scheduling, placement, preparation, and recovery according to the clinical characteristics of the scheduled procedure and the patient's medical needs, subordinating and synchronizing these processes to critical resources (step three). It was determined that a cost-benefit analysis and

CASE STUDY

approval by the executive leadership team were needed before the constraint was elevated (optional step four). A six-bed IR patient care unit was commissioned to be designed. The need for outpatients to be admitted to hospital care units for preparation and recovery and nonprocedure tasks occupying procedure rooms has been eliminated.

As a result of the ProcessVSA, use of existing IR and CT resources was enhanced, increasing Throughput and capacity. Quality of care and patient satisfaction were enhanced. The algorithm also served as a template for communicating with doctors' offices, patients, and nurses preparing or recovering IR patients on hospital units, thus preventing the primary root cause of bottlenecks in the value stream. Outpatient procedure cycle time was reduced by 40 percent, inpatient procedure cycle time was reduced by 20 percent, and CT capacity was increased by 50 percent.

to specifically identify the constraint, if not to perform the rest of the five focusing steps as well.

Documenting the Ideal and Future States

After documenting the current state of the process, the team then brainstorms about how the perfect process would be. Referred to as the *ideal state*, in designing it, the ProcessVSA team should assume that there are no barriers and that anything is possible within reason. This is where the team's creativity is particularly useful. Developing the ideal-state map should not take a lot of time and usually is limited to one hour. The purpose of the ideal state is to envision what the process could look like if all the non-value-added steps could be removed and flow were optimized. The ideal state typically has far fewer steps than the current state of the process.

By taking a look at this "perfect" process, the improvement bar is set high. If the team starts with the ideal state of the process as a point of reference and then thinks in terms of adding back as few steps as possible, the ideal provides a new paradigm for the improved process. This paradigm typically will involve removing more steps than without consideration of an ideal view or perspective. Dramatic, transformational improvement should not be expected if only the current state of the processes is considered with minor incremental tweaks. In some cases, teams considering the ideal state when designing the future state have been able to achieve the reduction of as many as half the total steps in the process.

The next step is to create a *future-state* process that represents the improved process the team actually plans to achieve over the next one to six months. Once the future-state map is developed and documented, the key opportunity bursts and constraints are identified, and a plan of action and milestones is set up to address each of them. Some of the improvements will be quick hits (also known as "just do its"), fixes that become obvious as the VSA is conducted and can be assigned to an individual to implement immediately. Very few improvements will involve a traditional project-type of effort. An example might be a change in software to fit with the new work practices. However, the major improvement impact can come from rapid improvement workshops focused on making substantial and fast improvements within the process in just one week. In addition, a plan is developed to manage the bottleneck, if there is one, and to address other constraints that impede flow. An example of current- and future-state maps for an emergency department process is given in Figure 6.6.

The future-state map is the team's vision of immediate or near-term improvements. The future-state map should be achievable in one to six months. After the ideal- and future-state maps are prepared, the team can move to the next phase, which is to identify the performance-improvement opportunities. Once improvement opportunities are identified, the team prepares an outbrief for executives.

Outbriefing the Event

The final task for the event is to prepare and deliver an outbrief. The audience, format, and content for a ProcessVSA outbrief tends to vary greatly across healthcare organizations. At a minimum, the ProcessVSA champion and process owner should be present at an outbrief. Depending on the impact of the ProcessVSA and the level of executive involvement in the operational aspects of the performance-improvement deployment, the outbrief may include the executive leadership team. Executive attendance at the outbrief is more common in the earlier stages of a deployment. The format of outbriefs is also highly variable. While the corporate standard for most presentations is the ubiquitous PowerPoint slideshow, it is not always the case. In some instances, the poster paper and sticky notes used in the

Current State   **Future State**

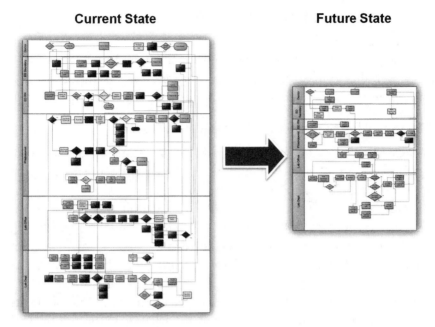

Figure 6.6 Example of current- and future-state maps.

event itself serve as the focal point of the outbrief. The content should tell the story and include the following elements:

▲ Why the event was conducted
▲ The event's findings
▲ The event's results

Post-event

Just because a performance-improvement event is over doesn't mean that there isn't work left to do. Real change happens after the event. The future state becomes a reality only when all action items are completed as planned. A ProcessVSA post-event roadmap appears in Figure 6.7.

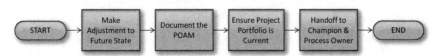

Figure 6.7 Post-event roadmap.

Making Adjustments to the Future State

In some instances, additional information may come to light after the event. Occasionally, changes may be driven by the comments during the outbrief. Whatever the source, the future-state process map is finalized—and transitions to becoming the new current state as changes are implemented.

Documenting the Plan of Action and Milestones

A *plan of action and milestones* (POAM), work plan, or whatever local version of the tool is used should be developed to document the path forward. It should address specific issues or actions necessary to carry out the process improvements recommended by the team. Any improvement actions that require new or follow-up activities should be included. Additional rapid improvement workshop and Six Sigma projects are not addressed as POAM milestones because they must be added to the organizational project portfolio and prioritized against other improvement opportunities. The POAM should include specific actions and requirements necessary to implement the improvements as delivered in the outbrief and approved by the champion.

Updating the Project Portfolio

It is common for additional improvement opportunities to be identified as part of the ProcessVSA. An example is when a changeover step has been identified as a problem, the solution is not obvious to the team, but the root cause is known. In this case, the problem should be documented as a future rapid improvement workshop and added to the project portfolio.

Handoff to Champion and Process Owner

When the entire package is complete, it should be handed over to the ProcessVSA champion and process owner for implementation.

Quick Hits

A *quick hit* is defined as an improvement initiative that produces a quantifiable savings or improvement as prescribed within the context of a performance-improvement activity, such as a Lean event or a Six Sigma project. Quick hits are usually the product of other performance-improvement activities, but some healthcare organizations will capture quick hits regardless of the initiating activity as a means to ensure all savings associated with performance improvement are captured. While many quick hits require little action other than to *just do it*, others can be quite complex. Quick hits vary in level of effort and cost but generally do not require additional analysis to determine their efficacy. Changes resulting from quick hits also should be within the approval authority and capability of the champion.

For more complex opportunities, the proposed improvements are documented in a *quick hit worksheet*, which is a simple tool to list each improvement and the person responsible for implementing it. A column for approval can be included if necessary. Quick hit worksheets do not require great amounts of detail. If a more formal action plan is needed, the champion will be responsible for its development.

Rapid Improvement Workshops

A *rapid improvement workshop* (RIW) is a focused, fast-paced, team-oriented event. The RIW is arguably the most adaptable and agile tool in an integrated performance-improvement toolset. Like many quality tools, the fundamental structure of an RIW is not new or unique to Lean. An RIW uses small cross-functional teams of carefully selected subject matter experts to solve a clearly defined problem for which the root cause is known, but the solution is unknown. This definition links RIWs to its origins in Shewhart's plan-do-check-act (PDCA), Deming's quality circles, Masaaki Imai's kaizen, and General Electric's workout.

The RIW is the best choice for many performance-improvement opportunities. Several common denominators are the reasons for the RIWs adaptability and enduring success:

▲ A short time frame, typically three to five days
▲ A narrow scope, a single problem, subprocess, or step in a process
▲ A clearly defined problem
▲ A small, empowered team of five to eight people who are intimately familiar with the process
▲ A skilled lead practitioner
▲ A standardized process for conducting the event
▲ A focus on work practices, not machinery
▲ An emphasis on creativity, not capital investment
▲ A focus on tangible, immediate results

Other names for an RIW include *rapid improvement event* (RIE), *kaizen blitz*, and *kaizen burst*. *Kaizen* is the Japanese word for "rapid improvement" or "change for the better" and was the vehicle for rapid-cycle performance-improvement endeavors within the Toyota Production System. The term *kaizen* encompasses both ProcessVSAs and RIWs. The difference is scope. In the book, *Kaizen Desk Reference Standard*, Raphael L. Vitalo and colleagues describe a kaizen that could require as long as six months to complete. Jeffrey Liker indicates that a kaizen blitz or point kaizen, focused on a specific process or event within a value stream, can be completed in as few as three to five days in *The Toyota Way Fieldbook*. While a ProcessVSA focuses on a process in its entirety, the objective of an RIW is to make a specific improvement in a narrow-scoped process.

The RIW model used in the integrated approach, while sharing origins and common denominators with PDCA and workout, does have some distinct differences. The addition of the find-organize-clarify-understand-select–plan-do-check-act (FOCUS-PDCA) strategy by the Hospital Corporation of America provided a link to organizational strategy and definition of the problem, according to Judith A. Schutt in the article, "Balancing the Health Care Scorecard." FOCUS-PDCA lacks a means to monitor and provide ongoing steady-state management of variation, and it does not address sustainment of improvements. General Electric's workout also lacks a robust control mechanism, as Dave Ulrich and colleagues criticize in the book, *The GE Work-Out*. The greatest difference between RIWs and a workout is the expected outcome. The deliverable of a workout is some recommendation(s) by the team regarding process improvements and a go/no go response from management. The team is not empowered to make the changes necessary to achieve the desired future state.

The RIW team uses existing available data to make swift improvements to a targeted problem or performance gap. Known root cause(s) and existing data are key differentiators between an RIW and a Six Sigma project and the reasons that an RIW can be completed in three to five days, whereas a Six Sigma project typically requires three to six months. For a Six Sigma project, a measurement system must be validated, and data must be collected and analyzed before a root cause can be determined. When chartering an RIW, process data such as that generated by VSA or system constraint analysis quantify the problem statement and are made available to the team early in the course of the event.

RIWs typically use a wide variety of tools to mitigate the seven deadly wastes of Lean described in Chapter 1 (i.e., overproduction, excessive inventory, excessive conveyance, unnecessary motion, waiting, defects, and extra processing) or to take action to mitigate constraints. For example, an RIW might focus on reducing batch size in cytology preparation, decreasing changeover time in patient examination rooms, implementing 5S in sterile processing, increasing Throughput in emergency department triage, or examining and managing constraints and bottlenecks.

The need for an RIW can be identified through several sources:

▲ SystemVSA
▲ ProcessVSA
▲ Six Sigma project
▲ Strategic gap analysis
▲ Key metrics/scorecard gaps
▲ Leadership direction
▲ Other RIWs

Several RIW events may be generated from any one source. Reducing flow time, increasing Throughput, or reducing defects is accomplished as a result of many RIWs. The RIW team establishes specific, measurable objectives to be accomplished during the event and at least one primary metric by which the success of the event will be evaluated. The scope of the RIW is narrow and discrete. This allows the RIW to be completed in five days or less. Some narrowly focused RIWs can be finished in several hours.

The lack of a standardized process is frequently identified as a root cause for performance issues. Additional analysis is not necessary to identify that standardization is needed, but the subject matter expertise and time commitment necessary to develop and document the standard process require that a team of subject matter experts representing all key stakeholders be convened in an RIW to develop and test the standard process.

An RIW also can be used to develop visual controls or other tools, such as standardized forms and templates, when the details of the solutions are not clearly understood. For example, a set of standardized admission orders would best be created in an RIW that includes the physicians who would be the primary users of the orders. Other likely candidates for an RIW are development of algorithms needed for pain management or mobility assessment, identification of the contents of supply kits or carts, and definition of the steps to implement an emergency action cascade for a full house census.

An RIW can be used to mitigate constraints. For example, a policy constraint prohibiting overtime may be identified in a CRT. Revising the policy could be accomplished with an RIW. Further analysis is not necessary to determine that the revised policy is needed, but structure, facilitation, and the appropriate subject matter expertise are necessary to create a policy that will be implemented successfully.

During the RIW, it is critical that team members are focused intently on the event. Leadership awareness and engagement are necessary to ensure that team members are able to dedicate time and attention to the event and to authorize and follow-through on recommended improvements identified by the team. The RIW champion is a division, department, or work cell leader with the authority to charter and empower the team. The lead practitioner provides direction to the team, performance-improvement subject matter expertise, and just-in-time (JIT) training to augment team members' knowledge and skills related to the use of performance-improvement tools and methods. The lead practitioner is responsible for event logistics such as scheduling, facilitating, and creating agendas for team meetings; for preparing the charter and reports; and for communication with the team and even the champion. Prerequisites of an RIW include

▲ Active leadership support and sponsorship
▲ Process mapped or clearly understood by team members
▲ Process data readily available
▲ Performance gap quantified
▲ Availability of team members
▲ Lead practitioner trained in performance-improvement tools and methods

Prior to initiating the RIW, the performance gap should be confirmed, the process must be clearly understood, and a root cause must be identified. Consultation with stakeholders, process owners, customers, and business leaders may be necessary to gather the information required to charter the RIW and to determine that there are no schedule conflicts, such as the absence of key team members or resources, or impending compliance audits, which would preclude a successful event.

Activities associated with the RIW are guided and directed by the charter. The charter includes a concise problem statement that clearly delineates and quantifies a single discrete problem. The business case describes the financial and/or customer rationale for undertaking the RIW and the benefits expected to be realized. A financial subject matter expert is consulted to estimate return on investment. The customer who is expected to benefit from process improvements resulting from the RIW is identified. A statement of the goal(s) of the RIW includes a quantifiable change in target process performance. Key event milestones are identified, and a timeline is determined to gauge team progress. Alignment with organizational strategy is validated and articulated. It is critical that the scope be sufficiently narrow to allow the team to accomplish objectives and milestones within the RIW time frame.

The robustness of an RIW makes it somewhat problematic to define a standard process. As described earlier, an RIW is used when the root cause is known and the solution or means to mitigate the root cause is the goal. The path toward solution identification generally is left to the practitioner. It is largely a matter of facilitating the team to the goal. An RIW is an event-based approach and will be addressed further in its three phases: pre-event, event, and post-event.

Pre-event

Pre-event preparation is crucial. An RIW pre-event roadmap appears in Figure 6.8. An RIW requires the focused dedication of team members for five days or less. Proper preparation by the lead practitioner and the champion is necessary to accomplish event objectives within the allotted time frame. Selecting an RIW champion, forming the project team, and chartering the RIW are all done similarly to the way they are done in a ProcessVSA pre-event. The data analysis done in a ProcessVSA is supplemented in an RIW by identification of at least one primary metric by which the success of the effort will be evaluated. An operational definition of the metric is determined and documented. Secondary metrics also may be defined to monitor the impact of process changes on related critical indicators such as safety and compliance. Baseline process performance and start and end points are also noted.

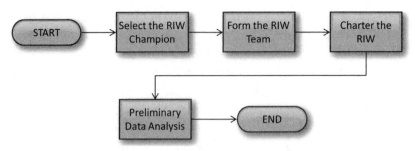

Figure 6.8 RIW pre-event roadmap.

Event

By their very nature, RIW events are intended to be a very robust approach to performance improvement. They can be applied to virtually any issue facing a healthcare organization. While the outcomes will vary based on the problem being addressed, an RIW involves a team of subject matter experts that is formed to focus on a specific issue. While conceptually this is easy to understand, the lack of a specific set of steps makes the application difficult to teach to new practitioners and leads to a high variation in approach.

Application of the Focused Facilitation Within an RIW

The process for facilitating an RIW can be standardized in such a way that it maintains its versatility, adaptability, and agility as the best means to solve a problem and create measurable, sustainable improvements in the least amount of time and at the lowest cost. The steps to facilitate an RIW are shown in Figure 6.9 and are listed below:

▲ **Focus the event.** The event charter is reviewed, and the RIW is officially launched. Ground rules are established and JIT training is provided. A *parking lot* list is set up to record issues that arise that are out of scope for the present event but which have merit and will be addressed later. Roles are clarified, and the event schedule is reviewed.

▲ **Evaluate the process.** The lead practitioner presents data, existing process maps, standard operating procedures or other process guidance, and any other relevant information to the team. The team assesses process performance and examines performance gaps. The difference between the current state and the future state is clearly understood.

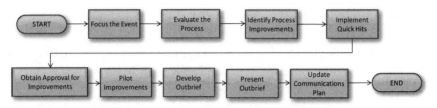

Figure 6-9 RIW focused facilitation roadmap.

▲ **Identify improvements.** The team brainstorms potential process improvements and assesses their feasibility and impact. Consensus is reached regarding the plan of action and prioritization of improvements.

▲ **Implement quick hits.** Improvements that do not require approval or capital investment and can be accomplished during the course of the event are completed.

▲ **Obtain approval for improvements.** If necessary, the champion and/or process owner review improvements that require approval, communicate requests to the appropriate persons or departments, and provide feedback to the team. Improvements requiring approval typically involve investment of resources or affect key stakeholders not represented on the team.

▲ **Pilot improvements.** Piloting or testing is necessary when the scope of the change is large or reversing the change could be difficult or costly. Acceptance for the change and support for improvements can be enhanced when the expected results and the practicality of the solution can be confirmed before full implementation.

▲ **Develop a plan of action and milestones.** A plan of action and milestones is developed throughout the RIW event and updated as action items are completed. The POAM includes a description of the task, the estimated date of completion, the owner or person accountable for completion of the task, the current status, and a column for notes.

▲ **Develop the outbrief.** The lead practitioner, with input from the team and feedback from the champion, develops a summary of the event that communicates the information essential for leadership and key stakeholders to understand why the event was conducted and what results were achieved. The presentation should be in a format that is appropriate for executive-level presentations and as brief as possible, including information in easy-to-read graphic form and accompanying handouts or appendices to provide details.

▲ **Present the outbrief.** The outbrief typically is presented by the lead practitioner and/or champion. The audience includes key leaders, team members, and any stakeholders affected by process changes. Team members should be recognized during the outbrief, and the audience should be provided with an opportunity to ask questions.

▲ **Update the communication plan.** The event communication plan is updated to include the results of the event and any other pertinent information. (Communications planning is discussed in Chapter 5.)

The lead practitioner applies traditional facilitation tools and techniques such as brainstorming, multivoting, affinity diagrams, and others as the means to accomplish these steps.

Application of DMAIC Within an RIW

Another method to standardize the RIW approach is to apply an abbreviated Six Sigma DMAIC, as shown in Figure 6.10 and as popularized by Michael George in the book, *Lean Six Sigma.* While it is used widely, there are several concerns or cautions that should be considered in applying this approach. The first is that DMAIC is a methodology to identify and analyze root causes. If the root cause is already identified, then the analyze phase is somewhat unnecessary. Another issue is that Six Sigma is a very structured methodology that emphasizes data and the application of statistical analysis. It can be confusing, especially for new practitioners, and lead to taking the same *abbreviated* approach to applying DMAIC in a full Six Sigma project.

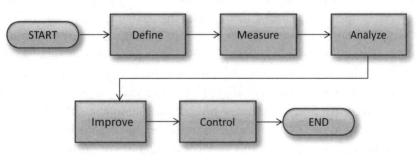

Figure 6.10 RIW DMAIC roadmap.

Application of Constraints Management Thinking Processes Within an RIW

What if there were a set of tools available that would be applicable across the full range of issues that an RIW tackles? Constraints Management has been around since the early 1980s. As much a philosophy as a methodology, its thinking processes are detailed in Chapter 2. Six Sigma uses data analysis as its source of rigor; Lean has the alignment with the Lean archetype; Constraints Management thinking processes use logical validity testing in an interactive process with the categories of legitimate reservation.

The categories of legitimate reservation are rules for scrutinizing the validity and logical soundness of thinking processes logic diagrams. Seven logical reservations are used:

▲ Additional cause reservation
▲ Causality existence reservation
▲ Cause insufficiency reservation
▲ Cause-effect reversal reservation
▲ Clarity reservation
▲ Entity existence reservation
▲ Predicted-effect existence reservation

The application of the thinking processes allows a healthcare organization to solve virtually any issue through a facilitative approach. While there are many possible ways to facilitate an RIW team to success, the thinking processes allow an organization to standardize an approach and teach a structured method. It helps practitioners to progress toward self-sufficiency more quickly than a less structured approach.

While there are many approaches to problem resolution that have been applied in these types of event-based efforts, the application of a single approach across virtually all types of opportunities reduces variation and ultimately improves both the efficiency and the effectiveness of RIWs. We promote the application of Constraint Management thinking processes tools introduced in Chapter 2. The roadmap to using the thinking processes within an RIW is shown in Figure 6.11.

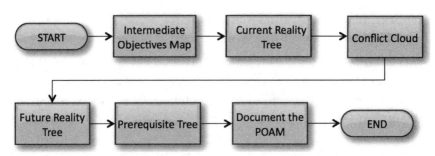

Figure 6.11   RIW thinking processes roadmap.

Post-event

The lead practitioner's responsibilities related to the RIW continue in the post-event, whose steps are identical to those of the post-event of a ProcessVSA. Issues captured in the parking lot are either referred to the appropriate party or resolved. A control plan is developed in which metrics and methods are established to monitor process performance over time and sustain improvements. The plan of action and milestones includes any necessary training of workers regarding process changes. The champion ensures that process improvements and controls are implemented as described in the POAM and control plan.

Once the improvements have been fully implemented, the process owner is responsible for validating the savings and return on investment resulting from the improvements with the financial subject matter expert. The communication plan is updated to include new information, such as process improvements implemented and savings realized. It is critical that this information be communicated to team members, stakeholders, and leadership after the RIW event has been concluded.

A summary of the RIW event is prepared by the lead practitioner and provided to the RIW champion that includes the following elements:

▲   Before and after performance of the targeted process
▲   Problem and root cause addressed
▲   Solutions evaluated
▲   Process improvements implemented or planned

The lead practitioner should document the RIW thoroughly so that the team's efforts and process improvements can be recognized and replicated in similar or related processes. Completion of the RIW is an opportunity to reward team members and celebrate success. This frequently overlooked step is critical to the continued success of RIW events as part of a performance-improvement deployment across the organization.

Six Sigma Project

Six Sigma projects apply many traditional performance-improvement tools within the Six Sigma five-phase DMAIC approach to produce statistically significant improvements in a process and real financial benefit to healthcare organizations. Selecting a Six Sigma project champion, forming the project team, chartering the project, and analyzing preliminary data are all done similarly to the way they are done in an RIW pre-event.

Apply the DMAIC Methodology

The DMAIC methodology includes the application of a full range of statistical tools yet recommends that it be implemented by teaching these statistical methods to workers throughout an organization. While the DMAIC methodology emphasizes the use of statistical tools, the strength is in the methodology itself.

In an article for the American Statistical Association, Roger Hoerl addressed how nonstatisticians can grasp the intricacies of these tools without undertaking the full coursework normally associated with statistical practitioners. Hoerl holds that the strength and success of the methodology are not in the rigor of the statistical tools but that the thoroughness of the DMAIC, "which provides a detailed, easy-to-follow, scientific inquiry approach," all but ensures success.

Reporting, Project Review, and Approval Process

Reporting and approval processes vary greatly among healthcare organizations. In many cases, Six Sigma projects cross organizational boundaries and directly affect the quality of the product or service received by the customer, whereas other process-improvement events generally affect the flow of the product or service. Additionally, Six Sigma projects generally take more time and a higher level of effort than VSAs and RIWs.

Reporting

Given these differences, Six Sigma projects are often briefed to the executive leadership team. While organizational norms for presenting to executives take precedence, the presenting practitioner should balance presenting the accomplishments of the project—the traditional *keep it simple* approach used in executive briefings—with his or her role as a change agent. A certain level of *technical content* should be included to demonstrate the application and strength of the tools.

Project Reviews

The phased nature combined with the cycle time of a Six Sigma project lends itself well to interim reviews, or *tollgates*, as they are commonly called. Across virtually all industries, practitioners provide *tollgate presentations* to their champions at the end of each phase of the five-phase DMAIC approach. These allow the champion to review progress and make course corrections as necessary.

Approval Process

The project champion should have an approval process for Six Sigma project recommendations just as they do for most Lean events. Occasionally, cross-functional projects are assigned a champion who does not have complete approval authority. While not the preferred approach, it recognizes that—while technically appropriate—senior executives generally delegate the role of champion even if he or she is the leader who has *positional authority over the scope of the process being improved.*

Balanced Scorecard

Measurement is the foundation of quality. It is said that if it can be measured, it can be managed. It is also said that a can of worms is still a can of worms even if you don't open it. The first step to improving a process is to measure and analyze the ability of the process to meet the needs of the customer.

When a performance-improvement project is conducted to close the gaps of a process's capability, team members are tasked with various action items with target dates. Performance cannot be improved until all action items of improvement projects are completed as planned. Since task owners also have their day jobs, giving priority to these action items becomes a major challenge. Regular follow-up meetings of team members are recommended along with frequent reminders in order to track progress, especially financial results.

A *balanced scorecard*, as described by Kaplan and Norton, is a valuable option in continuous performance improvement from a systems perspective. A balanced scorecard is compatible with a value compass, dashboard, cockpit, and data map, and in some organizations these terms are even synonymous.

The balanced scorecard is a tool and a process for tracking financial results while simultaneously monitoring the system's capabilities to meet customer specifications, key performance indicators, and critical success factors. A balanced scorecard is considered *balanced* when it includes financial and other indicators. The balanced scorecard is a performance measurement tool. When adapted for healthcare, indicators of effectiveness and efficiency, clinical quality, customer satisfaction, regulatory compliance, and learning and growth measure progress toward long- and short-term goals.

The balanced scorecard is a strategic planning tool that translates corporate vision and strategy into an integrated set of objectives. The balanced scorecard process is contiguous with strategic planning and budget development and provides a clear link to internal and external customers. The balanced scorecard must be created to optimize the efficient use of a system's valuable resources—leadership time and attention. It is critical to include only the *critical few*, not the *trivial many*, indicators necessary to monitor system performance. A hierarchy of indicators is detailed. This ensures that each level of management has precisely the information necessary to make decisions within its scope of authority.

In general, a balanced scorecard includes indicators divided into four perspectives or quadrants. This division reflects organizational vision, mission, and values and should not resemble an organizational chart. There are many examples to be found in the literature. When creating a balanced scorecard, it is important to benchmark the best both within healthcare and in other industries. A noteworthy benchmark for healthcare is described by the Institute for Healthcare Improvement (IHI). The IHI model includes whole-system measures (WSMs) divided into three dimensions: patient-centered, effective and equitable care, and efficiency. A fourth dimension, equity, is a stratification of WSMs by subpopulation.

The identification of perspectives or quadrants is a decision made by executive leadership as part of the strategic planning process and is as unique as the organization it is designed to serve. What is important is that it provides a compass for linking strategy to action and that it is communicated and *owned* at every level of the organization.

A balanced scorecard for a healthcare organization might include four perspectives—clinical quality, financial viability, customer loyalty, and operational effectiveness, as shown in Figure 6.12. Clinical quality would include measures of patient safety and clinical outcomes. Financial viability would include measures of financial strength and growth. Customer loyalty would include the results of net promoter score surveys for internal and external customers, patients, staff, and providers. Retention of critical staff, such as nurses and pharmacists, also would be included in a loyalty indicator in the customer loyalty quadrant. Operational effectiveness would include measures of compliance, staff efficiency, and management process capability. The balanced scorecard must be revisited and revised annually as part of the organization's strategic planning process.

The indicators at the executive leadership level represent the acme of a hierarchy of indicators that ultimately reaches the bedside and the loading

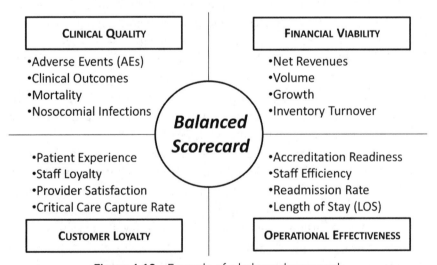

Figure 6.12 Example of a balanced scorecard.

dock. Every employee of the system knows how his or her performance affects the uppermost corporate indicators of the balanced scorecard. When the balanced scorecard is employed to its fullest potential, every department and division manager monitors performance relative to the indicators at his or her tier in the hierarchy. A detailed work plan defines the indicators and hierarchical relationships between tiers, providing operational definitions, targets, and ranges for red, yellow, and green status indicators. Online training and reference manuals provide guidance to users and ensure data quality. A software application translates raw data into graphic displays including trends and measures of variation. A portion of a sample work plan is shown in Table 6.1.

Table 6.1 System Balanced Scorecard Workplan

Indicators	Definition	Calculation
Clinical quality		
Rate of adverse events (AEs)	Inpatient AEs per 1,000 patient-days	Total number of AEs/total length of stay for all patient records reviewed × 1,000
Clinical outcomes	Clinical performance indicators	EWA of composite scores for core measures and EF-12
Mortality	Hospital standardized mortality ratio (HSMR)	Number of hospital deaths in acute care/number of acute-care discharges
Nosocomial infection rate	Rate of hospital-acquired infections	Infections/patient days × 1,000
Financial viability		
Net revenues	Revenues, cost	Total revenues – costs per DRG target
Volume	Inpatient and outpatient days	Days/target × 1,000
Growth	Increase in market share	% increase in market share/% projected
Inventory	Replenishment of inventory	Revenue/inventory
Customer loyalty		
Patient experience	Mean net promoter score (NPS)	Mean NPS response/number of patients surveyed × 100
Staff loyalty	Staff satisfaction and retention	Mean NPS response/staff/rate of staff turnover × 100

(continued on next page)

Table 6.1 System Balanced Scorecard Workplan *(continued)*

Indicators	Definition	Calculation
Provider loyalty	Mean net promoter score (NPS)	Mean NPS response/medical staff × 100
Operational staff loyalty	Mean net promoter score (NPS)	Mean NPS response/number of operational staff × 100
Operational effectiveness		
Accreditation readiness	Regulatory compliance	Mean % compliance with regulatory requirements
Staff efficiency	Staff per occupied bed	Full Time Equivalents (FTEs) per occupied bed
Readmission rate	30-day readmission rate	Number of discharged patients readmitted to the hospital within 30 days of discharge × 100
Length of stay (LOS)	Median LOS	Median LOS for targeted Diagnosis-Related Groups (DRGs)

In order to support performance-improvement efforts, the balanced scorecard is oriented toward improvement action. It provides a balancing mechanism by which opportunities for performance improvement are scrutinized and checked. Then, using data generated by control plans and statistical process control, the balanced scorecard monitors progress toward organizational, division, and departmental objectives. The balanced scorecard is a living entity that changes as organizational strategy shifts to accommodate an ever-changing environment. At any one point in time, the balanced scorecard reflects the condition of the organization and the gap that exists between the current state and a desired future state.

Generating Innovative Solutions

Breakthrough improvements require out-of-the-box thinking, innovation, and invention. None of the three methods, namely, Lean, Six Sigma, and Constraints Management, actually tells a performance-improvement practitioner what the new solution should be. Lean shows where the waste is and what slows down the flow, but then it is up to the improvement team to take the current-state map and decide what the new future state should look like. Similarly, in Six Sigma, statistical analysis tools allow the practitioner to narrow down the important few variables that cause variation, but it is up to the project team to generate solutions to control those variables in order to stay within specification limits.

Similarly, the five focusing steps of Constraints Management advise team members to exploit the system constraint after it is identified, but they do not say how. Again, it is up to the team to create solutions to get more out of the system constraint. If the thinking processes are used, developing injections is necessary based on the current reality tree to develop the future reality tree, and it is left to the improvement team to generate innovative solutions. If the team identifies a core conflict, it needs to be broken to generate win-win solutions. The team is expected to break one or more of the branches creating the conflict by creating innovative solutions.

Creating solutions is all about thinking differently in a way that creates value. The most frequently used tool to develop solutions is brainstorming. There are several more systematic and proven breakthrough-improvement tools. They can be broken into two main categories:

1. Techniques that psychologically stimulate creativity and inventive knowledge are included in the first category. These techniques change the thinking patterns and team attitudes but bring no additional knowledge into the innovation session. Examples of these tools include de Bono's six thinking hats; lateral thinking; directed attention thinking tools (DATTs); the substitute, combine, adapt, modify, put to other uses, eliminate, and reverse (SCAMPER) idea-generation tool; to name a few. These tools work best if the solution lies inside the experience of the team because they depend on team members' knowledge and their personal creative capability to generate ideas collectively.
2. The second category includes techniques that challenge psychological inertia and increase capability and knowledge. These techniques bring additional knowledge into the innovation session. The theory of inventive problem solving (TRIZ) contains numerous tools in this category.

Theory of Inventive Problem Solving (TRIZ)

TRIZ is based on an analysis of creative solutions of past challenges in different industries. It works great if the problem is complex or the solution lies outside the experience of the team. It allows organizational teams to achieve breakthrough improvements in a performance-improvement program. TRIZ tools can be used in a variety of areas but are mainly applied in the following five:

▲ Fact finding and defining the issue
▲ Problem understanding and analysis
▲ Idea generation
▲ Solution evaluation
▲ Acceptance of ideas and implementation

TRIZ History

TRIZ (pronounced "treez") is a Russian acronym for *teoriya resheniya izobretatelskikh zadatch*, which, when translated literally, means "theory of solving inventive problems" and is known commonly as the *theory of inventive problem solving*. Genrikh Saulovich Altshuller (1926–1998) created TRIZ. Altshuller introduced three underlying concepts that make TRIZ tools unique and different from other methods:

▲ Problem and solution patterns were repeated across different industries, products, processes, and services. The same fundamental solutions have been applied over and over again. TRIZ helps to find that standard problem, understand it, and applies its solution to a specific organizational problem.
▲ People are not born inventors. Innovation is a product of the human mind and can be improved using psychological techniques. To reach an *ideal final result* (IFR), or *ideality*, people reach for solutions that have all the benefits but none of the risk and cost nothing. To achieve free or idle resources within the current system, ideas are sought to optimize a solution.

The primary aim of TRIZ is to resolve contradictions between two opposing requirements on the same or differing objectives rather than accepting a tradeoff or compromise. The TRIZ community embraced Constraints Management tools, especially the conflict cloud. Integration of TRIZ with Constraints Management was introduced by Dr. David Bergland and has significant potential to progress the performance-improvement evolution.

Altshuller screened over 200,000 patents looking for inventive problems and solutions. Of these, 160,000 were basic improvements, which meant that they were applications of already known physical or technological principles. However, 40,000 were somewhat inventive solutions. One key finding he concluded from reviewing the patents was that consistent patterns of invention were used across different industries. Innovation was systematic, not random. Altshuller continued his research, and over 2 million patents were reviewed with the same findings. He concluded that innovation evolves through several levels. Altshuller posited five levels.

▲ **Level 1: Solution apparent**   A simple technical improvement. Requires no external knowledge.

▲ **Level 2: Small innovation**   Within a company—usually with compromise. Knowledge exchange—people transfer it, same industry

▲ **Level 3: Substantial innovation inside technologies**   Knowledge collaboration—customers/across industries

▲ **Level 4: Innovation**   Usually science outside technologies. Knowledge innovation—systemic management process

▲ **Level 5: Discovery**   Innovation and new science.

TRIZ Tools

TRIZ principles and tools can be applied in places where practitioners believe they will have the greatest impact on achieving the goal. For example, if idea generation is needed, TRIZ has a set of tools to accomplish this, such as identification and utilization of available/idle resources or seventy-six standard solutions. In general, TRIZ has tools for idea generation, combining, critiquing, and solution evaluation as well as problem understanding, identification, formulation, and categorization. There are numerous TRIZ tools and techniques. Listed below are seven of the more common tools. The intent of this listing is to briefly describe the tools and their applications. Additional readings will be necessary to gain a full understanding of these tools and their applications.

▲ **Ideal final result (IFR).** A basic concept of TRIZ is that systems evolve toward increasing ideality (functionality) and that the final destination is the IFR. It is a description of the best possible solution with no constraints to eliminate rework by solving the right problem the first time. Usually IFR is not an attainable goal, but when used correctly, it moves the team in the direction of a solution by overcoming psychological inertia.

▲ **Identification and utilization of available idle resources in the system.** The TRIZ definition of a resource is unique. It is all *positive*—also known as *useful*—and *negative*—also known as *harmful*—resources. Identification and utilization of available idle resources holds that one should strive to use available resources before introducing new resources into the system.

▲ **Forty inventive principles.** TRIZ is based on three major cornerstones—contradiction, harm, and ideality. The most effective inventive solution is the one that overcomes some contradictions. When a system has reached its peak performance, improvement of any features of a system can cause a conflict. There are two types of conflicts—technical and physical contradiction.

An example of a *physical contradiction* is where project managers need to set and maintain clear, stable priorities, but the very nature of many projects requires flexibility and changes. A *technical contradiction* might be where banking transactions are faster and easier but result in increased fraudulent transactions, such as money laundering.

The 40 principles are solution triggers—very general ideas of how to resolve a contradiction. This is one of the easiest TRIZ tools to use and the one most likely to result in good solutions easily and quickly.

▲ **System operator—nine windows.** A very simple but powerful tool where the context (system) is set up, and and the environment (supersystem) and all the details (subsystems) are defined. It is similar to looking at a dynamic presentation rather than a static image. According to system operator, we have to take into account not only the system itself but also its supersystem and subsystems. For each of these supersystems, systems, and subsystems, the past, present, and future also must be considered. As shown in Figure 6.13, this tool consists of nine windows that help to find the correct problem.

▲ **Functional analysis and trimming.** Functional analysis is an analytic tool that identifies the characteristics of important system components. It describes how these components functionally interact with each other and super- and subsystems. Functional analysis also helps to understand costs and how they contribute to or detract from the IFR.

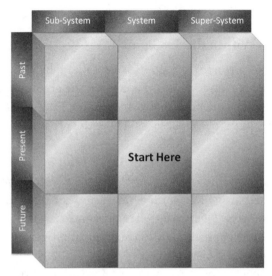

Figure 6.13   System operator—nine windows.

Trimming is an analytical tool, used to simplify the system, after identifying functional analysis diagram and/or table, by removing components with harmful effects to increase ideality. IFR usually contains fewer system components and simplifies the overall system.

▲   **Smart little people (also known as smart little creatures).** This method was developed by Altshuller in the 1960s as a psychological inertia-breaking tool through the use of overcoming expert terminology. It imagines a system with many clever small creatures that behave in the same way as the system. The team examines the problem details at the micro level.

▲   **Seventy-six standard solutions.** This is a general list of all recorded system model design solutions by science and inventors in patents. It is divided into five sections and shows all known ways to solve a problem. The five classes are as follows:

▼   Improving the system with no or little change

▼   Improving the system by changing the system—dealing with harm (prevent, transfer, and block)

▼   System transitions

▼   Detection or measurement of something

▼ Strategies for simplification, improvement, and cost reduction

TRIZ Applied Within the Six Sigma DMAIC

Six Sigma is well known to be a data-driven methodology. While the analysis of data is a crucial component of Six Sigma, the ability to apply creative thinking throughout the project also adds value. TRIZ creativity tools can be used throughout the five phases of a DMAIC project.

Define

▲ *Ideal final result (IFR) and ideality* help to determine the best value of a given metric in an ideal world of no waste where the proposed changes produce no harm. This is referred to on some charters as an *entitlement*. It also could be applied in project scoping, multigenerational projects, or defining success factors.

▲ The *system operator-9 window* provides nine perspectives on the problem to enhance the team's usual system-level perspective.

▲ *Identification and utilization of available/idle resources* in the system enable you to select the right team to work on the problem and evaluate standard operating procedures (SOP).

▲ *Functional analysis and trimming* ensure that the team understands the system components and how they work together.

▲ If the team identifies physical or technical contradictions in the system to meet the critical to quality (CTQ), voice of the customer (VOC), voice of the business (VOB), or to resolve conflicts from the roof of the house of quality (HOQ) in the quality function deployment (QFD), then the *40 inventive principles* can be applied to improve or eliminate technical contradictions.

Measure

▲ Similar to the Define Phase, utilization of the *system operator-9 window* provides nine system-level perspectives.

▲ *Functional analysis and trimming* ensure that the team understands the system components and how they work together.

▲ *Identification and utilization of available/idle resources* in the system enable the use of resources when conducting sampling, capability analysis, or measurement system analysis (MSA).

▲ If the team identifies physical or technical contradictions in the system when conducting sampling, capability analysis, or measurement system analysis (MSA), then the *40 inventive principles* can be applied to improve or eliminate technical contradictions.

Analyze

▲ *Identification and utilization of available/idle resources* in the system enable performance-improvement teams to identify potential root causes of the problem.

▲ The *smart little people* tool aids in the understanding of processes at the micro level to validate the root cause of the problem. It helps the team to overcome psychological inertia induced by the use of specialized terminology.

▲ *Function analysis and trimming* identify insufficient functions, contradictions, and the source of harmful actions.

Improve

▲ *Identification and utilization of available/idle resources* in the system help the team to create a future-state process map, develop an implementation plan, and communicate the solution to stakeholders.

▲ The *smart little people* tool aids in the understanding of processes at the micro level to develop an implementation plan. It helps the team to overcome psychological inertia induced by the use of specialized terminology.

▲ *Function analysis and trimming* help the team to create a future-state process map.

▲ The *40 inventive principles* give the team a way to generate solutions to eliminate the contradiction and find optimal settings—not compromise.

▲ The *76 standard solutions* give the team a way to generate solutions.

Control

▲ *Identification and utilization of available/idle resources* in the system help the team to implement solutions, develop a control plan, and establish a process monitoring system.

▲ The *system operator-9 window* helps the teams in making decisions at the right level. It can be used to decide what level solution and what time-scale solution to apply.

▲ The *40 inventive principles* give the team systemic benchmark methods from patient knowledge bases to reduce the risk of implementation.

CASE STUDY

TRIZ

A rapid improvement workshop (RIW) was conducted to address coordination of patient care in the emergency department (ED) of a community hospital. The RIW was the result of a ProcessVSA that had focused on the reduction of turn-around time (TAT) for STAT laboratory tests.

During the ProcessVSA, a value analysis of the process revealed that 30 percent of the delay in TAT was due to the order-to-collect time: the time from physician entry of the order to collection of the specimen. A lack of coordinated access to the patient by ancillary services (i.e., laboratory, radiology, respiratory, etc.) was identified by root-cause analysis to be a key contributor to delayed STAT laboratory orders. About 25 percent of the time, the phlebotomist would respond to the ED to collect the specimen only to discover that the patient was not in the bed. The phlebotomist then would seek out the nurse caring for the patient to determine where the patient had been taken and when he or she was likely to return. If the patient had been taken, for example, to radiology for a computed tomographic (CT) scan, the phlebotomist then would go on to collect other specimens, often on other hospital units. On return later to collect the specimen, the phlebotomist might find that an electrocardiogram (ECG) was being performed or a respiratory treatment was being given, causing further delay.

The goal of the patient care coordination RIW was to reduce order-to-collect time by coordinating access to the patient. It was immediately apparent to the team that a new process was required. It was agreed that it was the inherent role of the ED nurse to coordinate ED patient care. The order in which specimens were collected, diagnostic studies conducted, and emergent treatments administered should be determined by the needs of the each patient, the tests and treatments ordered, and nursing logic. Some radiologic studies take only a few minutes to complete, whereas others take 20 minutes or longer. A specimen takes just moments to collect, but common laboratory studies require an average of 28 minutes of processing. If care was coordinated

CASE STUDY

properly, the patient could be taken to radiology while his or her complete blood count (CBC) and coagulation parameters are being processed in the laboratory. Some means of communicating with ancillary providers was needed.

The ED had an electronic whiteboard that displayed the location and some status information about patients but did not display the information necessary to coordinate patient care. While brainstorming solutions to the problem, the team became mired in frustration related to "fixing" the electronic whiteboard's software. To generate innovative ideas, the facilitator introduced the TRIZ tool called *ideality*. Ideality takes advantage of resources in the system, such as nursing expertise, and resolves contradictions.

The *ideality checklist* guided the team through a process to define an ideal final result (IFR). An IFR does not introduce any harm into a system or increase the system's complexity. It preserves all the advantages of the existing system while eliminating the disadvantages.

The solution was a simple, reliable, real-time tool that allows the ED nurse to communicate the appropriate order of care to ancillary services. The tool included a feedback loop so that if the laboratory was given access before radiology transported the patient to a Magnetic Resonance Imaging (MRI) machine, radiology would know that the specimen had been collected.

As shown in Figure 6.14, a simple signal flag created from office supplies and found objects was created and piloted in the ED. Order-to-collect time for STAT laboratory tests decreased immediately to 16 minutes, a 66 percent improvement. These savings translated directly to ED length of stay, a key cost driver for the hospital.

Feedback from the ED staff also was collected. The flags were used for several days until the staff could clearly articulate how the flags support the process and how their function could be improved, if not constrained, by obvious design limitations. This information then was used to create a set of specifications for upgrades to the ED whiteboard software.

TRIZ tools allowed the team to see beyond the problem and the presumptive solution ("fix" the software) to the ideal solution. A simple,

CASE STUDY

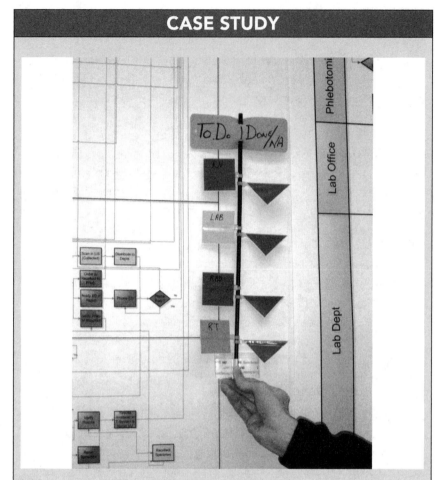

Figure 6.14 Signal flag.

manual interim solution made an immediate impact on the process and ultimately produced the model and specifications necessary to make appropriate changes to the software, as shown in Figure 6.15. As a result of clearly communicating the needs of the staff to the software developers after piloting the solution, the ED whiteboard software now functions in a way that supports patient care and works very effectively for the ED clinical staff.

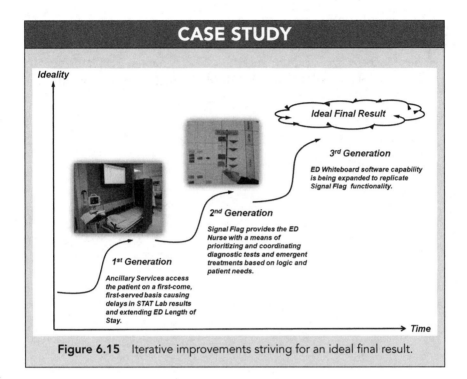

CASE STUDY

Ideality

Ideal Final Result

3rd Generation

ED Whiteboard software capability is being expanded to replicate Signal Flag functionality.

2nd Generation

Signal Flag provides the ED Nurse with a means of prioritizing and coordinating diagnostic tests and emergent treatments based on logic and patient needs.

1st Generation

Ancillary Services access the patient on a first-come, first-served basis causing delays in STAT Lab results and extending ED Length of Stay.

Time

Figure 6.15   Iterative improvements striving for an ideal final result.

TRIZ is a breakthrough improvement set of wide-ranging tools and techniques, an innovation method, a philosophy, and a way of thinking. TRIZ tools can provide a sequential, multilevel approach that helps professionals from all walks of life to develop both strong creative solutions and skills. When people encounter TRIZ for the first time, some tools can be overwhelming. Therefore, we recommend that its philosophy be understood prior to applying the tools. It is only after the philosophy is understood and each tool is mastered that practitioners should move on to using new tools.

Conclusion

In order to close performance gaps, action must take place to change the process. Every methodology has a range of tools designed for this very purpose. Practitioners trained in—or biased toward—a single set of tools will risk less than optimal results, suboptimizing the system, taking too long to achieve the results, or not being able to sustain the gains. By employing an integrated toolset along with a detailed deployment plan, practitioners will be able to realize exceptional results. Next, Chapter 7 explains how to sustain those phenomenal gains that the performance-improvement team worked so hard to achieve.

CHAPTER 7

Sustainment

"What we can or cannot do, what we consider possible or impossible, is rarely a function of our true capability. It is more likely a function of our beliefs about who we are."

—TONY ROBBINS, AUTHOR

Performance-improvement sustainment is an ongoing state whereby a healthcare organization is continuously improving its processes with minimal external support. This path to self-sufficiency requires organizational commitment over an extended period of time. At the highest level, a performance-improvement deployment is approaching sustainability when the program is contributing more to the organization than the resources it uses. In addition to quantifying deployment efficacy and ensuring that project results are being realized and replicated whenever possible through the use of sound deployment metrics—addressed in Chapter 5—leadership must be proactive in the development of organic capability.

Organic Capability

While it is a fairly common practice to use external consulting support as a temporary measure until organic capability is developed, leadership must pursue internal capability aggressively. *Organic capability* means a cadre of performance-improvement practitioners throughout the organization taking actions to close performance gaps.

Program Oversight

The next level addresses how those performance-improvement resources are managed. The program management office concept was discussed in

Chapter 6. While a healthcare organization may have invested in the training and development of a decentralized cadre of practitioners, the program management office—under the guidance of the deployment champion—must ensure that their efforts are supportive of organizational strategies and that methodologic rigor is maintained. In many instances, the deployment champion has not progressed to the advanced practitioner level necessary to provide the requisite technical support and oversight. Champions are neither required nor expected to be advanced practitioners. This drives a requirement to have at least one advanced practitioner assigned to the program management office.

Other roles of the mature program management office include management of the project portfolio as well as scheduling training and development for new and existing practitioners. Succession planning for current practitioners is also needed to ensure continued performance-improvement capability despite turnover.

The practitioners dispersed throughout the organization generally focus their efforts locally. All action, even if globally aligned, is local. Centralized full-time resources—assigned to the program management office—also lead more complex cross-functional or enterprise-level projects. While there is an obvious requirement for at least one centralized advanced practitioner, depending on the size of the healthcare organization, additional resources may be required. The centralized practitioners are advanced practitioners capable of running multiple projects, mentoring others, advising leaders throughout the organization, and in many instances delivering training. Another critical component of the program management office is to maintain the deployment metrics and advise the executive leadership team on performance improvement.

Program Assessment

As the deployment progresses, it is essential that it be evaluated for overall efficacy. The primary evaluation tools are the deployment metrics established during the plan phase. Assuming that a comprehensive set of tools was developed, no additional data/feedback may be necessary.

One area that generally requires additional scrutiny is customer/stakeholder satisfaction and perception. An internal survey can be used to determine internal customer satisfaction. It is recommended that any assessments applied during the assess phase be reapplied periodically to monitor progress. While the utility of periodic change readiness assessment is widely practiced, the follow-on assessment of performance-improvement maturity is often overlooked.

While the criteria that establish a prima facie case for program maturity are readily evident—strategic alignment, deployment planning, opportunity/resource management, organic capability, benefit realization, and so on—the perception of the leadership team (target respondents for the maturity assessment) is often assumed or ignored. While the actual progress through requisite events/deliverables is important, the perception of progress by the executive leadership team is equally important. If a deployment is apparently hitting all the checkpoints, yet members of the executive leadership team respond negatively, corrective action is necessary.

After-Action Reviews

An *after-action review* (AAR) is a structured and reflective process whereby the participants of an event, incident, or operation examine how the event was managed in a nonincriminating manner with the objective of organizational learning, extracting learning points, and proposing improvements through a constructive and participative group dialogue. Over time, AARs—first applied by the Israeli Defense Force and later popularized in the U.S. Army—have become a powerful tool for organizational learning.

While AARs involve a relatively simple process, they require careful planning and attention to the organizational culture to ensure an open dialogue and a safe environment. This did not take place overnight in the U.S. Army. Figure 7.1 shows an example of the AAR process. Each review is different, and it is more important that the intent be met than the letter of the process flow.

The U.S. Army "Training Circular on After-Action Reviews" provides the specific point for conducting AARs:

▲ AARs are conducted during or immediately after each event.
▲ They focus on intended training objectives.
▲ They focus on soldier, leader, and unit performance.
▲ They involve all participants in the discussion.
▲ They use open-ended questions.
▲ They are related to specific standards.
▲ They determine strengths and weaknesses.
▲ They link performance to subsequent training.

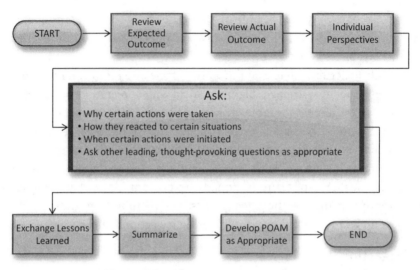

Figure 7.1 After-action review process.

AARs are a simple, low-cost means to enhance future performance, encourage team behaviors, and promote organizational learning. Failure to implement this methodology in a performance-improvement deployment may have a negative impact on the overall efficacy of the deployment. AARs are useful not only for individual events and projects but also for entire performance-improvement deployments.

Succession Planning

It is important to recognize that trained practitioner turnover within their own staff is inevitable. In many industries, it is a common practice that senior practitioners should serve as full-time performance-improvement practitioners for two to three years. Even if a more permanent model is adopted, turnover is inevitable—whether the move is upward or outward. With the skills and organizational knowledge gained, it is a waste when these valuable resources leave the organization. Career paths should be developed for these practitioners to grow within the organization—transitioning from performance improvement to the operational side of the organization so that the investment can continue to reap benefits. With this ongoing turnover in skilled practitioners, the performance-improvement training program also must be ongoing. This drives the development of organic training and mentoring capabilities. Not only must these departing practitioners be replaced, but healthcare organizations also must begin developing advanced practitioners.

Mentoring Revisited

The development model for senior performance-improvement practitioners is the traditional apprentice-journeyman-master model, as discussed in Chapter 5. Depending on the type of deployment—greenfield, revitalization, or new heights—the role of the mentor changes, as seen in Figure 7.2.

This is based largely on the recognition that true mastery cannot be gained through didactic learning alone. As discussed previously, there are options regarding where a healthcare organization gets the advanced practitioners needed to initiate mentoring in the early stages of a deployment. If mentoring is contracted, it should be provided on a decreasing scale offset with increasing levels of autonomy and a subsequent assumption of responsibility by in-house practitioners. A timeline should be established.

Greenfield
- Blank canvas for building a mentoring program.
- Select known high-performers for initial projects.
- Achieve rapid, initial success and buy-in across the organization.
- Mentoring resources are generally not available internally.

Revitalization
- Make compromises to fit mentoring program within established infrastructure.
- Focus on identifying and revitalizing projects with strategic importance.
- Acquire professional mentoring support if internal resources don't exist.
- Renew/build commitment from a cadre of champions.

New Heights
- Stable, sustainable program exists at an average or higher level of maturity.
- A formal mentoring program enables the organization to evolve into a higher level of performance excellence.
- Program focuses on balancing knowledge transfer and ROI.

Figure 7.2 The role of mentoring in a performance-improvement deployment.

Training

For many deployments, initial training is outsourced to a performance-improvement consultancy. Recognizing the need for follow-on mentoring and project support, care should be taken when selecting the training source. Many people and groups provide training and then leave organizations on their own for follow-on mentoring.

As in-house advanced practitioners gain skills, a transition plan should be developed to allow the training to be done internally. In many instances, this is accomplished incrementally by absorbing responsibility for champion training first and then progressing incrementally through the levels of complexity—initial practitioner training second and then more advanced topics/courses. In many deployments, training is the last activity to be transitioned to internal resources. One often neglected aspect critical to practitioner development is the skill of change management. Accordingly, we recommend that the training of this vital soft skill not be ignored.

Integrated Change Management

> "To improve is to change; to be perfect is to change often."
> —WINSTON CHURCHILL

In today's competitive and highly volatile economic environment, change is the rule, whereas the steady state is momentary and uncertain. Change management must be embedded in the technical transformation that is taking place—a process within a process. Successful continuous performance-improvement deployments must address change management throughout the deployment process. The devil is in the dynamic details. How to implement a change program successfully is critical when dealing with another confounding variable—the erratic changes of human behavior reacting to changes. The most successful organizations have people who must learn to continuously adapt to change.

Change happens, unabashedly. Whether it is planned or unplanned, positive or negative, change is the new norm. In healthcare, change has transmuted to an oxymoron, a constant—technological changes, regulatory changes, legislative changes, economic changes, demographic changes. Sometimes these changes are not incremental but are revolutionary, affecting every part of the system. Change is either imposed or is proactive. When W. Edwards Deming cynically said that "change is not necessary; survival is optional," it was never more true than it is of healthcare today. When asked to describe the pace of change in healthcare today, a nurse wearily replied, "Change is all there is."

Proactive change, such as a performance-improvement deployment, is intended to move the organization in a positive direction. Performance improvement, by design and by definition, is a change initiative. While all change does not lead to improvement, performance improvement inevitably requires change. With the barrage of change that is already pummeling healthcare, performance-improvement initiatives may be perceived by overworked and overwhelmed staff as the next-last straw. Thus change-management skills and methods are fundamental to any performance-improvement endeavor. Performance-improvement practitioners are expected to act as change agents and change leaders. They need to be equipped, empowered, and trained to facilitate and manage change. Any successful performance-improvement deployment will be founded on change-management principles and methods.

But deliberate, proactive change is not easy. Harvard Professor Kotter estimated that 70 percent of change efforts fail. Peter Senge, who was named "Strategist of the Century," noted that failure to sustain significant change recurs over and over again despite substantial investment of resources, including talented and committed people. Only 41 percent of projects successfully meet project objectives related to time, budget, and quality. Fifteen percent are abandoned or fail completely. This results in lost investments averaging more than 134 percent of the original cost of the project—with no results.

Healthcare is an industry that is especially resistant to change. The Institute of Medicine (IOM) noted a 17-year lag between the publication of research and its impact on patient care. This delay in applying evidence-based best practices to product or service delivery is unimaginable in other industries.

Barriers to Change

Barriers to change tend to be cultural or organizational. In a *Financial Times* article, Carolyn Pexton identified common organizational barriers to change in healthcare. Some of these barriers are among the following:

▲ Cultural complacency, resistance, or skepticism
▲ Failure to communicate
▲ Poor strategic alignment
▲ Lack of ownership and accountability
▲ Insufficient leadership support
▲ Micromanagement
▲ Overburdened workforce
▲ Inadequate systems, processes, and infrastructure
▲ Decentralized organizational structure (i.e., tribe mentality)
▲ Lack of control plans to measure and sustain results

Healthcare has unique cultural implications for change management. One factor that makes change especially difficult to manage in healthcare is the fact that physicians, in general, do not work for hospitals. This is one reason that physician resistance is identified as the most difficult barrier encountered by healthcare change leaders. Organizational silos prevail in healthcare on both the macro and micro levels. Departmental silos include nursing, medicine, patient safety, risk management, finance, human resources, and so on. Within each department, microsilos exist: critical care, surgery, medical surgical, home health, and hospice. Each silo has its own culture, incentives, and information systems.

While a customer-focused service industry would seem to demand a matrix organizational structure, integration and interoperability are rare in healthcare. *Interdisciplinary* is an industry buzzword, but until recently, true inter-anything was practically nonexistent. Inexorable economic forces and impending healthcare reform are driving changes. According to an article in the *Journal of Health Service Research and Policy* by Tim Scott and colleagues, healthcare organizations that emphasize group affiliation, teamwork, and coordination are more likely to implement quality improvements successfully than those with more formal structures and reporting relationships. Performance-improvement practitioners must be capable of identifying and mitigating barriers to change.

Success Factors

Certain factors have been linked to successful change endeavors. Change management is more art than science. Much of the success of change efforts depends on the soft skills of communication, negotiation, and influencing.

In an IBM study, top-management support was identified as the most important factor for successful change (92 percent), followed by employee involvement (72 percent), honest and timely communications (70 percent), and a corporate culture that motivates and promotes change (65 percent). The U.S. Army identified eight success factors for change management:

▲ A sense of urgency
▲ A clear and shared vision
▲ Engaged leadership
▲ Communication
▲ Involved stakeholders
▲ Enhanced change capability
▲ Project integration
▲ Performance and organizational alignment

General Electric (GE) identified reasonable expectations, definitive boundaries, project execution structure, and clear roles as factors contributing to successful change. Hard factors can be measured and are the technical aspects of change management. A Boston Consulting Group study identified a consistent correlation between the outcomes (success or failure) of change programs and four key factors—project duration, the time between project reviews and milestones, performance integrity, the skills and capabilities of project teams, the commitment to change displayed by both senior executives and affected staff, and the additional effort demanded of staff to cope with change.

Successful change efforts (including performance-improvement deployment), projects, and events require a consistent attention to and skilled application of both soft and hard change-management skills. An integrated approach to performance improvement is especially effective in that these skills are embedded in training and practice.

Change-Management Tools and Methods

The change-management tools used by various models include strength, weakness, opportunity, and threat (SWOT) analysis; stakeholder analysis; in frame/out of frame force-field analysis; SIPOC; 15 words; Approvers-resources-members-interested-parties (ARMI); Goals-roles-process-inter-personal (GRPI); and communication planning. These tools are not unique to change management but have been used for strategic planning, team development, performance-improvement, and other business transformation endeavors for decades.

The thinking processes of Constraints Management are also used to overcome resistance to change. As shown in Figure 7.3, this can be accomplished by systematically addressing nine layers of resistance or nine steps to buy-in, as described by Efrat Goldratt-Ashlag in her chapter about it in the *Theory of Constraints Handbook*. Achieving buy-in (agreement about what to change, what to change to, and how to make change happen) is the key to overcoming resistance to change and successful change initiatives. Each of the three questions must be addressed separately and in turn before buy-in (agreement on the problem, the solution, and the implementation) can be achieved.

The first three layers of resistance are based on disagreement about the problem. The first layer of resistance denies that a problem exists, hence

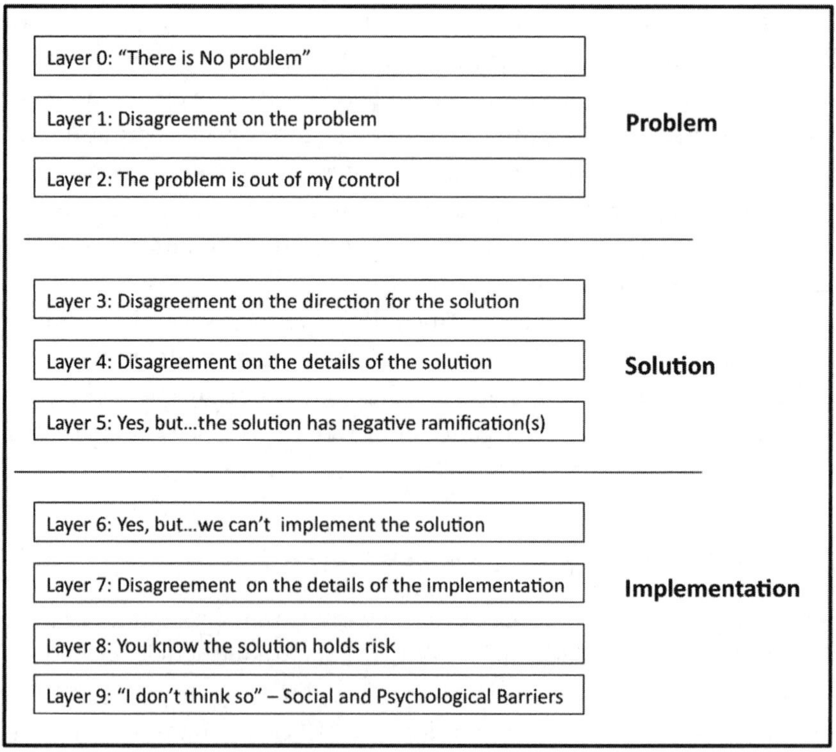

Layer 0: "There is No problem"	
Layer 1: Disagreement on the problem	**Problem**
Layer 2: The problem is out of my control	
Layer 3: Disagreement on the direction for the solution	
Layer 4: Disagreement on the details of the solution	**Solution**
Layer 5: Yes, but...the solution has negative ramification(s)	
Layer 6: Yes, but...we can't implement the solution	
Layer 7: Disagreement on the details of the implementation	**Implementation**
Layer 8: You know the solution holds risk	
Layer 9: "I don't think so" – Social and Psychological Barriers	

Figure 7.3 Layers of resistance to change.

layer zero. Nothing will change until there is agreement that a problem exists or that there is an opportunity worth pursuing. The best approach to peeling back this layer is to listen, challenge assumptions, and provide information. Until there is agreement that a problem exists, there is no possibility of buy-in.

The first layer of resistance is disagreement on the problem. This may be the result of different perspectives or roles. There may be a perceived lack of understanding. Empathy is key to address this layer of resistance. Thinking processes tools such as the conflict cloud and current reality tree are used to address this layer of resistance. The second layer of resistance is based on the assumption that the problem is beyond an individual's control. This is an especially difficult layer to overcome and may require taking the matter to a higher level of authority. Again, dialog may uncover erroneous assumptions and sources of empowerment.

The second three layers of resistance are based on disagreement about the solution. The third layer of resistance is disagreement about the direction of the solution, positive or negative, more or less. As discussed in Chapter 2, the conflict cloud is the thinking processes tool generally used to determine and to sell the direction of the solution. The fourth layer of resistance is disagreement on the details of the solution. This is an opportunity to think *outside the box* of your own perceptions. The future reality tree is used to address all of the Undesirable Effects. The fifth layer of resistance is the "Yes, but . . ." concern (often warranted) that the solution could have negative consequences. *Negative branch reservation* recognizes the value of input from those with concerns about unintended consequences and is the means of creating a good solution that solves the problem without causing significant new ones.

The last three layers of resistance are based on disagreement about implementation of the solution. The sixth layer of resistance is another "Yes, but . . ." concern that the solution can't be implemented owing to impracticality or other substantial obstacles. The prerequisite tree or strategy and tactics tree, for larger projects, identifies obstacles and map the means to circumvent them, either in parallel or in sequence. The seventh layer of resistance is disagreement on the details of the solution, the "Who does what?" and "What comes first?" In order to peel back this layer, the *why* must be made apparent. The transition tree conveys the rationale for each step in implementation. The eighth layer of resistance is the inability to convince the individual that the results outweigh the risk. Changing the risk-benefit equation is necessary to motivate change. Listening to objections and pausing to address them adequately should move the individual toward buy-in. If not, he or she may be "stuck" in a previous layer, and some reassessment is necessary.

Finally, it must be considered that resistance to change may be motivated by factors unrelated to the problem or solution at hand but is the manifestation of social and psychological barriers. This final level of resistance, layer nine, is the last frontier to achieving buy-in and can be addressed only through building relationships and effective communication. Identifying external factors as early as possible will provide an opportunity to alter the approach and address resistance without blame.

The key is to use the tools as part of a standardized, consistent approach that integrates the principles and methods of change management and project management with performance improvement. Our approach integrates change management into a seamless deployment-focused approach consisting of five interventions.

The first intervention in any change initiative is to assess readiness for change. As described in Chapter 4, we use a 5 × 5 change-readiness assessment to measure an organization's readiness for change in five important constructs:

▲ Communications
▲ Culture
▲ Leadership
▲ Organization
▲ Skills readiness

This evaluation is used as part of the assess phase, and the deployment plan identifies specific approaches to mitigate any gaps.

The second intervention is to gain everyone's attention. This can be done by creating quick results to kindle employee involvement in support of the change. The results must ensure consistency and honesty among the leaders, as well as from the leaders to the organization. Leadership must clearly define and model how to relate to each other, to customers, to stakeholders, and to all employees. Leaders also must identify strategic levers and carry out bold actions to wake up the organization to create a change strategy that reflects the desired culture.

We encourage the early application of process-based value-stream analyses and rapid improvement workshops as a means to realize quick results. Additionally, these activities tend to be both highly participative and visible. When combined with an effective execution of the communications plan and well-planned participant recognition, the likelihood of buy-in is greatly increased.

The third intervention is to build the momentum. This can be achieved by creating and promoting individual and team modeling through performance-improvement initiatives. Champions provide real-time observation, feedback, monitoring, and course-correction measures for teams in action. Team leaders can create partnerships between team members for two-way coaching. Executives can hold large group meetings focused on real-time activities for the organization's transformation. Successful execution of the communication strategy should create multiple vehicles by which stakeholders can see and, if possible, become part of the momentum. Progress, breakthroughs, stories of success, and desired behaviors should be celebrated. The communication strategy must support changing the mind-set.

The fourth intervention is to sustain and reinforce. The deployment plan should show a clear path forward. Properly developed and communicated, the deployment plan is a roadmap to sustainment. By following this roadmap, leaders are demonstrating commitment and reinforcing positive behaviors. Leadership may establish rewards for mind-set and behavior change, relationship improvements, and so on. The organization can hold periodic celebration events that provide team building for intact teams or new teams. Opportunities to reward/recognize employees who support change should be actively sought out.

Finally, the fifth intervention is perhaps the most vital—integration and strategic alignment. Our integrated approach provides a means to address this critical need. We recommend that all key aspects of the existing organization be analyzed, including structures, systems, processes, policies, and overarching goal. Accountabilities are assigned at the appropriate levels. For example, certain policy or market constraints may require that the strategic plan be revisited, whereas other actions can be taken immediately in the form of quick hits. All projects must reflect a direct linkage to the organization strategy and goals. In addition, resources to initiate improvement actions should be prioritized based on that alignment as well as impact on core drivers identified through the system constraint analysis. Additional strategic-level action might include a redesign of the succession-planning criteria, new hire criteria, or any other components of the organization to integrate/align with the desired performance-improvement culture.

Benefits and Return-on-Investment (ROI) Validation

Performance-improvement deployments need to be assessed in terms of benefits realized on a regular basis to ensure the viability of the program. Until recently, the primary rationale for undertaking performance-improvement initiatives in healthcare was *to do the right thing*, and any financial benefit resulting was appreciated as a fortuitous side effect. There is a preponderance of evidence that better-quality care costs less and that performance improvement is certainly the right thing to do. But a powerful motivation for performance improvement in healthcare today is financial viability. Evaluation needs to include the cost of building, maintaining, and upgrading the infrastructure of a performance-improvement program as well as cost-benefit analysis of individual projects.

Deployment Planning for ROI

The processes and infrastructure necessary to support the appropriate estimation and validation of project and event benefits are established in the early phases of a performance-improvement deployment. Achieving an ROI begins with aligning performance-improvement endeavors with organizational strategy articulated and defined in the assess phase. Strategic imperatives are identified, and projects and events are selected to ensure that performance-improvement efforts are directed toward those opportunities with the greatest potential for a financial return. This is first and foremost the responsibility of the executive leadership team. A system-level perspective of the organization and of internal and external forces affecting strategic decisions is necessary. An advanced performance-improvement practitioner with deployment planning expertise and experience guides the team to set a course most likely to consistently achieve positive financial results.

During the plan phase, the deployment team establishes the processes and practices by which performance-improvement project and event benefits will be estimated and validated. These processes are documented in standard operating procedures (SOPs) and applicable policies. Critical issues to be addressed by policy include the time frame for crediting project benefits, calculation of project costs and ROI, and credit for subsequent benefits resulting from replication. Roles and responsibilities are defined. Financial metrics against which to assess deployment success are developed. Training and references provided to performance-improvement practitioners, champions, and executive leadership include definition of project and event benefit categories and translation of operational process improvements to financial returns. Tools and templates are developed and standardized to ensure that processes are effective and efficient. Key terms and calculations are clearly defined. Financial estimation and validation tasks are included as expected and necessary steps in the charter, review, and closure of performance-improvement projects and events.

The guidance of an advanced performance-improvement practitioner during deployment planning is critical to demonstrating project and event benefits. While each deployment is unique, there is a core set of deliverables that must be created in advance of the first project or event chartered and often before the first performance-improvement practitioner is trained. Templates and samples provided by a deployment mentor significantly reduce the time and effort required to create critical documents such as the benefits calculation worksheet and SOPs. Providing a novice deployment team with benchmarks and best practices allows the team to craft and customize processes and practices that meet deployment deliverables while taking full advantage of existing infrastructure and considering their organizational culture. Expert deployment planning guidance also ensures that the team avoids common pitfalls and creates the best conditions for deployment success, including financial returns that meet and exceed leadership expectations.

Roles and Responsibilities

During the early phases of the performance-improvement deployment, the chief financial officer (CFO) must be involved in executive leadership training and deployment planning activities. More on the role of the CFO in financial estimation and validation appears at the end of this section.

The deployment leader should be made keenly aware of the potential failure modes associated with lack of financial leadership and all the elements necessary to support a robust process for estimation, validation, tracking, and reporting of financial benefits. The deployment leader performs a gatekeeper function, maintaining a project and event opportunity portfolio and ensuring that only projects and events that meet the selection criteria established by the executive leadership team are chartered. As the deployment matures, the deployment leader tracks, monitors, aggregates, and reports the results of performance-improvement projects and events, including financial benefits. As project and events are chartered and completed, financial data are aggregated by the deployment leader into a deployment benefits workbook (or a database) from which the ROI for the performance-improvement deployment is continuously calculated. Any deviation from the anticipated path of returns should be addressed according to a remediation strategy articulated during deployment planning.

The Process for Estimation and Validation of Performance-Improvement Benefits

Estimation of the potential for an ROI for a performance-improvement project or event occurs initially when the opportunity is identified and added to the opportunity portfolio. Most executive leadership teams identify ROI as a prioritization criterion during deployment planning. Once the opportunity has been identified as a potential project or event, a financial subject matter expert is consulted for an initial evaluation of the potential for an ROI. If the potential exists, data are collected to estimate the anticipated return. If not, the opportunity is not considered an immediate priority for performance-improvement efforts. It is the prerogative of executive leadership to override the process at this point. Should an opportunity present such a strategic urgency that the rationale for addressing the issue exceeds any anticipation for an appreciable financial benefit, the rationale should be carefully documented during the chartering process.

The role of a financial subject matter expert (SME) or quality analyst, sometimes called a *money belt*, is essential to any performance-improvement deployment. Those who will function as money belts are trained in performance-improvement methods so that they fully understand their role and responsibilities, including the estimation of potential ROI for performance-improvement opportunities, identification of data needed to estimate and validate project and event financial benefits, translation of operational improvements to financial benefits, monitoring and adjustment of estimates throughout the project or event life cycle, and calculating and validating the financial benefits and ROI of completed projects and events.

The financial SME collaborates with the project or event champion to categorize and link costs and benefits to the appropriate budget line item for organizational accounting purposes. The financial SME functions as an ad hoc member of the performance-improvement project or event team, attending team meetings only when financial subject matter expertise is needed and requested by the performance-improvement practitioner or champion. The financial SME reviews the current estimate of cost/benefit, is a part of every project tollgate or review, and his or her sign-off is a necessary condition to project or event progression to the next phase.

The role of the performance-improvement practitioner with regard to estimating and validating financial benefits begins during creation of the project or event charter. By clearly articulating a problem statement that links performance gaps to a business case, the basis of financial benefit calculations is established. The project goal—some improvement in process capability, as evidenced by one or more clearly defined metrics such as cycle time or percent defect—then is translated into financial terms. The performance-improvement practitioner and members of the performance-improvement team collect the process data needed to calculate financial benefits and ROI. The performance-improvement practitioner creates and maintains the benefits calculation worksheet for each project or event. The worksheet identifies anticipated savings by category and associated costs, recurring and nonrecurring. Careful documentation of operational improvements and resources is necessary, including time invested, to provide the information necessary to calculate project and event benefits and ROI accurately. When completed, data from the worksheet are aggregated by the deployment champion into a deployment benefits workbook from which the ROI for the performance-improvement deployment is continuously calculated.

Once finance has defined the data points needed to estimate project or event benefits, it is generally the responsibility of the performance-improvement practitioner leading the project or event to collect the data necessary to estimate the anticipated benefit to be achieved. The business case described in the project or event charter by the champion and the performance-improvement practitioner defines the link between operational improvements anticipated and financial results. A project or event goal, in operational terms described by the performance-improvement practitioner, is translated to financial terms by the money belt. This resulting calculation articulates the anticipated financial benefit identified by the project or event charter.

As the project or event progresses, estimates of financial benefit often evolve. The charter and tollgate reviews document changes as the process is better understood. As additional data and information become available, they are provided to the money belt, and estimates are refined and updated. At the close of the project or event, the operational results are compared with the goals articulated in the charter. The costs of any improvements, such as personnel, equipment, or software enhancements, are deducted for a net ROI. This figure, calculated by the money belt, is then "booked" by the performance-improvement deployment leader as the official estimate of project or event financial benefit and documented in project and event portfolio tracking systems. The process owner monitors control metrics for a predetermined period of time, generally two to six months, to ensure that process capability demonstrates sustained improvement. When the validation period defined by SOPs has been completed, the performance-improvement practitioner and process owner provide the money belt with the data necessary to validate the ROI. The project or event financial benefits then will be documented by the deployment leader in the deployment benefits workbook reported to executive leadership, included in deployment metrics, and credited to an ongoing calculation of deployment ROI.

The improvement-opportunities benefit estimation and validation process flow appears in Figure 7.4 and is described as follows: First, the deployment champion collects improvement opportunities and consults with the financial SME, who determines whether there is a potential ROI for each opportunity. Next, the executive leadership team prioritizes the improvement opportunities, taking into account overall ROI and other factors in strategic alignment with the organization's goal (e.g., quality of care, patient safety, staff satisfaction, regulatory compliance). The deployment champion then updates the opportunity database according to the priorities set by the executive leadership team. If the opportunity is addressed and has a potential for ROI, then the financial SME uses the

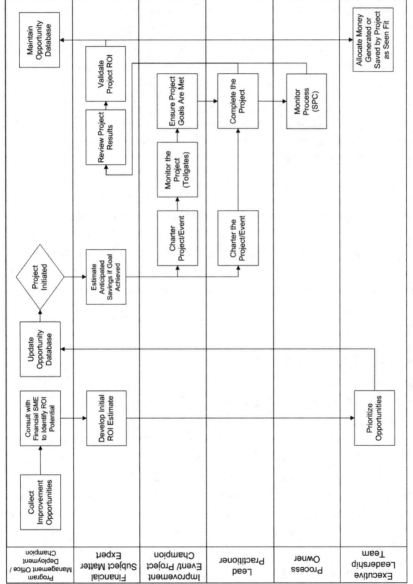

Figure 7.4 Improvement-opportunities benefit estimation and validation process flow.

257

estimated anticipated savings and revenue generation as the baseline to determine whether the financial objective of the improvement has been achieved.

After the ROI has been estimated, a champion for that improvement opportunity, alongside a green belt or black belt, charters the project or event. The project/event champion monitors the tollgates of the improvement effort to ensure that the lead practitioner and team are completing all related goals successfully and provides assistance, if needed. A review of the current estimate of cost/benefit is included in every project tollgate or review. The champion verifies that anticipated process improvements and associated financial benefits are aligned with organizational strategy in such a way that there is a clear line of sight between the endeavors of the performance-improvement team and strategic imperatives. Once the improvement effort has been completed, the process owner monitors the improved process, preferably using statistical process control (SPC). The financial SME reviews the results and validates the ROI of the completed improvement effort. The outcome and important data related to the event or project are then entered into the improvement-opportunity database by the deployment champion. In the meantime, the executive leadership team decides how to allocate money generated or saved by the project to the benefit of the organization and communicate the benefits widely.

Categories of Benefits

There are two general categories of benefits to be achieved by performance-improvement endeavors: operational and financial. *Operational benefits* typically cannot be linked *directly* to dollars either saved or generated and are often called *soft savings* or *operational improvements*. Examples of operational improvements include improved productivity in terms of decreased cycle time and lead time, increased output, increased patient safety, or reduced space utilization. Improvements in availability, safety, security, elimination of defects, and satisfaction and quality of life are operational benefits. So are increases in recruitment and retention, staff development, growth and competitive advantage, and environmental improvements such as reduction of energy usage and hazardous waste generation. Some operational benefits are associated with collateral financial benefits, but many are not and are thus called *soft savings*. A common factor in hospital financial analyses is the emphasis to decrease costs.

A hospital CFO recently told us, "The only way we can make money is to save money." This assumes that there are no opportunities to increase revenue. While cutting costs can have an immediate impact on the bottom line, financial managers should do so without missing the opportunities for growth and revenue increases. Even some federal agencies started tracking revenue generation separate from performance-improvement activities. Accordingly, financial benefits include

▲ Revenue generation
▲ Cost savings
▲ Cost avoidance

Financial benefits that can be linked directly to an impact on the bottom line are often called *hard savings*. These savings are permanent, quantifiable reductions in cost that can be linked to specific budget line items and can be removed from the budget. Cost savings include elimination or reduction in nonlabor costs such as equipment or supplies, contracted services, or overtime. Cost savings also include the reduction or elimination of full-time equivalent staff positions.

To make sure that an organization's staff understands that performance improvement is not about layoffs, we recommend the adoption of a policy to never eliminate positions as a result of gains achieved through performance improvement. Instead, we suggest the allowance of reduction of staff positions by natural attrition and only if protective capacity is not needed. Layoffs are never a preferred option and can become an insurmountable obstacle to a successful deployment if terminations becomes synonymous with performance improvement. To the contrary—an organization's policy never to cut staff positions owing to performance improvement enhances the motivation of participants in improvement efforts and engenders their invaluable support. Employees can take comfort in knowing that their efforts will not put them out of a job.

Cost avoidance is a permanent cost reduction that cannot be subtracted from an existing budget line item. This includes savings necessary to meet existing budget reductions or to unbudgeted items such as overtime or equipment maintenance cost. A common type of cost avoidance results from the prevention of adverse events such as accidents, noncompliance, or nonconformance. The costs or penalties for such events thus are avoided, but the savings cannot be attributed to any specific customer or account.

Revenue generation is achieved only through billing for new or additional services or products rendered. This includes revenues generated by new services, increased utilization of existing services, and increased collections for services provided. Financial benefits are the primary objective of performance-improvement projects and events in many cases.

Calculating ROI

There is no other industry in our nation's economy that experiences the level of financial complexity that characterizes healthcare. One of the greatest challenges to measuring ROI for healthcare quality is assigning value to improvements that do not yield savings in cash or for which improvements in one level of the industry or organization result in savings in another. Dlugazc notes an inappropriate linkage between healthcare finance and operations in his book *Value-Based Health Care: Linking Finance and Quality*. Calculations of project and event ROI vary from organization to organization and state to state. Since many hospitals and healthcare organizations are not-for-profit, this means that "the budget is a means to an end, a necessary condition, not the goal," as Dettmer noted in this book *The Logical Thinking Process*. Financial calculations such as operating margin, return on total assets, net present value, rate of return, and so on are the same as for for-profit organizations.

While some standard definitions exist, the calculations used to estimate and validate project and event benefits and deployment ROI should be consistent with established organizational accounting practices and language in order to be clearly communicated and credible. Financial SMEs are familiar with the equations that comprise a profit and loss statement.

Financial benefits are usually annualized, and the proportion of savings to be attributed to one year over another should be clearly defined by SOPs and policy. A conservative approach to ROI calculations is best. Failure to validate financial benefits has a demoralizing effect on practitioners and can irrevocably damage the credibility of the deployment. In general, investment ratio is calculated by dividing annual benefit by total cost. This reflects a need to focus on Throughput decision support, which is fundamental to Constraints Management, as opposed to traditional cost accounting.

It is critical that any calculation used to demonstrate financial benefits of performance-improvement projects or events be validated by finance. The best approach is to limit performance-improvement practitioners to providing operational improvement data to finance and using the subject matter expertise of a financial specialist to make financial calculations.

Optimizing ROI

There are three ways to maximize ROI—lower the investment, increase the returns, and reduce the time necessary to achieve results. Lowering the investment can be achieved by selecting the right projects and scoping them appropriately; by assigning the right practitioners, properly trained, mentored, and motivated; and by engaging in rigorous project management. Returns can be increased by selecting the right people and clearly defining their roles and responsibilities, selecting the right projects, and using the appropriate performance-improvement method. The time necessary to achieve results can be reduced by ensuring that practitioners are trained and supported properly. Other components of maximizing ROI include applying the appropriate performance-improvement methods and project-management techniques and scoping projects appropriately. All these conditions are set by a properly developed and executed performance-improvement deployment plan. Once the conditions are set, strategic decisions can be made and adapted as necessary to optimize ROI.

Early in GE's historic deployment of Six Sigma, the company performed a benchmarking study and regression analysis of factors influencing long-term company value and ROI. Strategic drivers such as market share, labor productivity, and capacity utilization were identified and linked to financial targets and project selection. The Institute for Healthcare Improvement (IHI) has performed a similar analysis for healthcare. The IHI uses Noriaki Kano's "three key aims" approach to defining value in a model for a balanced strategy of quality and value initiative. The resulting diagram is similar to that used by GE and identifies five primary drivers for cost savings through waste reduction in healthcare—clinical quality, staffing, patient flow, supply chain, and mismatched services.

Ronen and colleagues describe a process for identifying value drivers and the use of focusing tools to evaluate the relative potential of key drivers to add value and difficulty of implementation. This approach is more comprehensive and complex than the IHI model. The IHI model provides a focus for healthcare cost reduction in general, whereas focused operations management, based on Constraints Management, provides a means of selecting the best focus for performance-improvement initiatives that will deliver the greatest value in terms of increased top-line growth and bottom-line cost reductions.

Consistently adhering to a process similar to the one illustrated in Figure 7.4 will ensure that financial expertise is available when it is needed. Benefits of financial expertise include, but are not limited to, the following:

▲ Operational improvements will be translated appropriately to financial benefits.

▲ Financial calculations will be accurate and meaningful.

▲ Estimates of project and event benefits will be reasonable and realistic and based on established organizational accounting practices.

▲ The financial results of performance-improvement projects and events will be validated by finance and will be credible.

▲ The performance-improvement program will be measured and monitored in terms of financial ROI, with projects and events selected deliberately to bend the curve.

▲ Deployment objectives will be achieved.

▲ Reporting will be aligned, and deployment and organizational leaders will be able to articulate the value of the performance-improvement deployment to the organization.

▲ Performance improvement will be recognized as a highly effective means to an end (fiscal viability) and not just one more thing to do.

Role of the CFO

The CFO is a key stakeholder and major player in any performance-improvement deployment. The failure modes described earlier can be linked directly to lack of involvement and engagement of the CFO and his or her team. In 2006, Zinkgraf summarized the financial function in a Six Sigma deployment as "creating and validating financial results" and identified two categories of financial roles—providing support throughout projects and substantiating end-of-project savings/benefits. Project support includes qualifying project opportunities, identifying leverage opportunities, validating process measurement proposals, verifying dollar benefits as goals, characterizing or categorizing financial impact, and providing ongoing project financial-improvement evaluation. Substantiating savings/benefits includes authentication of project financial results.

Unfortunately, according to Dlugacz, many hospital CFOs do not clearly understand the relationship between delivery of care and clinical outcomes, the financial impact of poor outcomes, and the financial implications of inefficient processes. Maureen Bisognano of the IHI compared the involvement of healthcare CFOs in quality-improvement efforts with those of companies such as GE, Alcoa, 3M, and Johnson & Johnson. She noted that "the CFOs of these companies understood that the surest way to organizational success in terms of revenue, margin, and reputation was high quality." While Bisognano identifies recent advances in the involvement of CFOs in quality and highlights examples of committed financial leadership at Thedacare, Magee-Woman's Hospital, and Cincinnati Children's Hospital Medical Center, the level of engagement of CFOs at these organizations does not represent the norm.

As the person responsible for communicating the financial condition of the organization to hospital leadership, including the board of trustees, the CFO's involvement and engagement are critical to deployment success and credibility. Strategies to engage the CFO in quality and performance improvement include sharing a common agenda, speaking a common language, and taking a personal role, as Maureen Bisognano discussed in her article entitled, "Engaging the CFO in Quality." Educating the CFO and finance team is a deliverable of the plan phase for which there can be no compromise. Otherwise, a promising deployment may demonstrate impressive operational results and yet be terminated or suboptimized because cost/benefit analysis fails to demonstrate an appreciable ROI. This disconnect is particularly discouraging when the operational improvements have been achieved and validated. When CFOs are not engaged and debriefed appropriately during deployment planning, practitioners are left to translate improvements in process capability and efficiency into financial terms that can be credited to their endeavors without success.

Common Failure Modes

Making the commitment to invest in a performance-improvement deployment should be undertaken with the same degree of due diligence and trepidation as any capital investment. Training, developing, and supporting performance-improvement practitioners; investing and empowering performance-improvement teams; and championing and chartering performance-improvement projects and events all cost money. When the decision is made to launch a performance-improvement deployment, there are clearly articulated business reasons for investing in performance improvement, and there is an expectation of a return on that investment, often in a very short time frame. When the deployment fails to deliver or (just as important) *to document* the anticipated results, enthusiasm wanes, practitioners become discouraged, and deployment credibility disintegrates. Many of the "failed" deployments cited in the literature accomplished impressive operational results, at least initially. But because they failed to document a credible positive impact on the bottom line, those results did not figure favorably into a cost/benefit analysis of the deployment. Leadership support and resources dried up, practitioners moved on, and performance improvement became yet another "flavor of the month" that had lost its savor.

Whether intentional or accidental, the inflation of project or event savings and ROI is just as deleterious to a performance-improvement deployment as the failure to link operational efficiencies and performance improvements to financial benefits. There are several reasons inflation is likely to occur without the appropriate guidance and controls. Performance-improvement practitioners generally do not have a background in accounting. They are trained to calculate the operational improvements achieved from eliminating waste, managing constraints, and reducing errors. Translating these operational improvements into financial terms is beyond their scope of expertise. They may not understand or have access to the financial data necessary to calculate the cost of implementing process improvements. These costs may include personnel, software or hardware, and capital expenses that must be deducted from gross savings to calculate a net project or event return. Deployment metrics that link financial returns to measures of practitioner performance might provide an incentive for practitioners to overestimate or inflate the financial benefits associated with projects or events. Rigorous financial auditing processes ensure that gains are sustained and send a clear message of accountability to the organization.

Replication

In order to maximize ROI, replication should be a formal part of the performance-improvement work plan. Successful replication strategies make sharing and transfer an integral part of everyday work so that they are a natural part of work activities and not an afterthought. The same applies for replication in performance-improvement efforts. One way to integrate replication into the performance-improvement process is to make identification of replication opportunities part of the project deliverables. The literature suggests that successful transfer of information for best practices and replication should be both a *push* and a *pull* effort. The bottom line is that this is *advertising*. A product won't sell if no one knows about it. Similarly, gems cannot be replicated if no one knows about them. Cultural changes will not take place if no one knows about them, and so on.

At the start of all performance-improvement events and projects, practitioners should examine past and ongoing initiatives to determine which of those activities—their methods, findings, recommendations, results, and so on—can be leveraged in the current performance-improvement activity. Questions to ask at this stage include "What has been done in terms of methodologies and results in other initiatives that can be leveraged for this project?" "How can I adapt those methodologies or results for this initiative?" and "What lessons can I learn from other projects to make this one more efficient and effective?"

During the final phase of a performance-improvement activity, practitioners should identify replication opportunities for the results of their current activity. They should specifically ask the questions "Is this replicable?" "Who can benefit from it?" and "How can I help make it happen?" At completion of a performance-improvement activity, the person(s) responsible should formally inform potential business units/personnel about the resulting replication opportunities. Follow-up should take place to see if the informed party has assessed the opportunity and, if so, how promising? And if not, why not? This may involve working with the informed party to help assess the opportunity, secure funding, and adopt the change. When reviewing the literature associated with replication, it quickly becomes apparent that it is as much a change-management process as a performance-improvement process.

Another layer of replication is benchmarking with external organizations. Benchmarking can be done outside just a single organization; it also can occur with other healthcare organizations. Benchmarking outside one's industry also can be of use to realize solutions that have been undiscovered within the healthcare field.

Impact of Replication on Performance-Improvement Benefits

By now it should be apparent to all that performance improvement is a capital investment. The decision to proceed with an implementation that will realize the same results that were *paid for* once with a decreased subsequent investment seems to be obvious. The effort expended on the initial project can be viewed as *sunk costs* that are not recurring in subsequent replications. In an article by managers at Ford Motor Company, the authors state that they have been averaging close to 10,000 replication efforts per year, generating a value of $1.25 billion.

An article about a project-management software solution that supports replication states that there is a 12:1 ROI for replications. It states that each replication requires half the cost of a full project. The cost of each replication is given as 20 percent of the original project cost. It should be noted that there are two different types of replication. While the literature sometimes treats them synonymously, the preceding examples were referring to *replication of solutions.*

Replication of Solution   This is the most common and most efficient type of replication. An example of a solution replication is where a performance-improvement project was convened and successful. As an example, a project may be completed at one hospital of a multihospital system. The solution, while designed to meet the needs of the original hospital, may well be applicable to other hospitals in the same system. While minor adjustments may be required to account for local nuances, implementation time and costs generally are much lower because initial project work has been completed. An additional benefit of solution replication is that it increases standardization between work units or facilities. This enables staff to move between them with minimal transition difficulties.

Replication of Project   In some instances, the complex transactional healthcare processes may make direct replication of solutions impossible. In these instances, *replication of the project* should be considered. An example of project replication is where a performance-improvement project has been completed within a specialty clinic. Significant results are realized, but the clinic operates at only a single location. While this specific type of specialty clinic is unique, perhaps its problem is not.

CASE STUDY

Solution Replication

Within a military healthcare system, the cumbersome and lengthy credentialing process for contracted healthcare providers resulted in increased costs, difficulties in staffing critical positions, and delayed appointment availability. The current process did not meet the needs of internal and external customers.

Using Six Sigma DMAIC methodology, the project team investigated the credentialing process workflow variances. Lack of standardized tracking sheets, misaligned competency requirements, lack of user-friendly credentialing checklists, and broad questions on current medication usage and external verification of nursing competencies were identified as critical contributing factors. Implementing tracking sheets and credentialing checklists, aligning competencies, and rewording standard questions resulted in decreased credentialing cycle times. Improvements were statistically validated through hypothesis testing.

The project team implemented tracking sheets and credentialing checklists, aligned all competencies to one standard, and developed new standard questions that resulted in decreased credentialing cycle times with corresponding increases in sigma level and realized annual financial savings of $789,000.

The project results were briefed to the executive leadership team, which, after some dialogue, determined that the solution was applicable across the entire healthcare enterprise. Subsequently, they directed that the solution be replicated across the enterprise. On replication, financial savings are projected to reach $113 million.

Another clinic may be facing the same issues, but owing to significant differences in the process, the root causes of the problem can be different. In this case, the project may need to be run at the second clinic to determine the root cause. Much of the initial project planning, data collection or at least data source identification, measurement system analysis, and voice-of-the-customer research already may be accomplished in the initial project and can be applicable across clinics for the subsequent project(s). This would have a positive impact on the project cycle time and most likely allow for faster implementation of a solution unique to the second clinic.

Another example would be when the Pareto principle is applied and the scope of a project is reduced to focus on one customer group or error type—or any other segmentation. On project completion, the subsequent project to address the next-highest contributor should proceed more smoothly and rapidly.

Replication Within Military Healthcare Organizations and Other Large Systems Performance improvement between the military healthcare system and the Veterans Health Administration (VHA) have so much in common, and there is so much further potential in their collaboration. Each of their performance-improvement programs can be taken to new heights

CASE STUDY

Project Replication Case Study

A medium-sized public healthcare system was experiencing a high missed appointment rate in its dental clinic. Since the root cause of the missed appointments was not known, it was decided to apply the Six Sigma DMAIC methodology to address the issue. Analysis revealed that the largest attributable factor to missed appointments was a single client segment. The probability that this type of client would miss his or her appointment was predictable. Therefore, it was determined that *overbooking* certain appointments within the schedule was appropriate. While the behavior of this segment of the client population could not be changed, appointments in the schedule were filled, and utilization of the clinic improved significantly without any impact on patient satisfaction.

While other clinics also were experiencing problems with missed appointments, the executive team, in conjunction with clinic-level SMEs, were uncertain that the root causes were the same across clinics. As a result, a decision was made to replicate the project at other clinics. While the root causes did indeed show differences, the time necessary to complete the replicated projects was approximately half the original.

with each other's help. While these organizations have some differences, they also share many similarities in their approach to quality improvement as well as their overall focus on healthcare. The replication of projects goes beyond simply sharing best practices and affords the opportunity for future advances that can be mutually beneficial to both the military healthcare system and the VHA. The combination of the VA and military healthcare systems, jointly applying performance-improvement methodologies, can improve the performance of both systems and the quality of care provided to the military, their families, and the nation's veterans dramatically.

The military and VA healthcare systems have a great deal in common. They focus on providing world-class medical care and treatment to active-duty military, their families, and veterans. They are dedicated to ensuring that compassionate, cost-effective, and injury-free care is provided to all eligible patients. For this care to remain the very best possible, continued and highly focused improvement efforts must be made to constantly assess all healthcare processes for potential improvements. Performance improvement is a proven, reliable, and sufficiently robust methodology to improve those processes. However, it will continue to require top-down, executive-level support and commitment; all levels of hospital personnel must be involved, and sustainment of the improvement efforts must be monitored continually. The great news is that the early efforts in the military and VA medical treatment facilities clearly demonstrate that it works. There is enormous potential for both systems to jointly share best practices and then replicate their successes. The quality and effectiveness of patient care clearly will benefit from these efforts.

Taking Performance Improvement to the Next Level

The fundamentals of change management apply internally to a performance-improvement deployment. The economic environments, customer requirements, and even changes in culture and leadership drive business and organizations in different directions from year to year. In addition, performance-improvement methodologies and tools, as well as technology, are evolving very rapidly. As the business continues to change focus and new tools provide even higher performance, application of the organization's performance-improvement efforts must change with them.

In order to keep a performance-improvement effort alive and a viable part of a business, the focus must change to keep pace with the need. This may mean training master practitioners and mentors in a number of best-practice methodologies that are applicable to new objectives.

Introducing Constraints Management into Lean and Six Sigma Cultures

The evolution of performance improvement has been made possible by visionaries who took risks. They pushed the boundaries for new tools and methodologies for higher performance. It also takes patience. Introduction of a new method or tool into an industry where it never has been tried before sometimes takes years before it is accepted and used widely. If a new method or tool gives a major competitive advantage to an organization, there is reluctance to share success stories with the outside world. On the other hand, many organizations do not want to risk their resources on an unproven methodology or whose success stories are not available in the public domain. They want to hear what will it take to implement in their environment, along with the cost of implementation, the risks, and how fast they can see benefits. New methods require not only resources for training, but most important, major success stories also are needed to obtain buy-in.

In 2002, one such visionary, Dr. Gary Kaplan, CEO of Virginia Mason Medical Center, decided to implement Toyota Production System principles, also known as Lean thinking. He encountered formidable resistance, and some physicians even left the center. However, almost a decade later, that bold move of introducing the Lean methodology made Virginia Mason Medical Center one of the industry leaders. Virginia Mason knew what other hospitals are just now starting to realize: Performance-improvement methods need to evolve quickly to keep up with the business challenges in today's economy with spiraling costs of healthcare. Virginia Mason was not the first healthcare organization to apply Lean. As reported in 2000, the University of Pittsburgh Medical Center's isolated application of the Toyota Production System in healthcare provided some encouragement. With such successful results as reduced rates of nosocomial infections and diminished patient wait times, Dr. Kaplan saw the promise of what could be done with Lean in healthcare.

The term *Lean* was coined to describe the Toyota Production System during the late 1980s at Massachusetts Institute of Technology (MIT). Two decades later, its applications in healthcare began. Six Sigma's adoption in healthcare was not as protracted, but it still was almost a decade after Motorola introduced it. Even though Six Sigma was disclosed by Motorola in 1987, its widespread use did not start until Jack Welch decided to implement it in 1995 and made it a part of GE's DNA. And it didn't hurt that Welch was very vocal about the benefits of Six Sigma too.

Constraints Management in healthcare is finally gaining momentum, almost three decades after Goldratt introduced it in *The Goal*. Even in manufacturing, Constraints Management is not widely implemented yet. It took nine years for Boeing Integrated Defense Systems to fully adopt the critical chain project-management solution of Constraints Management owing to the radical cultural change it required.

There is some speculation on why Constraints Management took so long to gain traction within industry. Here are some possible reasons:

▲ It requires major paradigm shifts in the opposite direction of common practices, which some may find counterintuitive or an affront to established methods. Examples of generally discouraged practices include

▼ Balancing production and service lines

▼ Batching units

▼ Using cost per unit, cost-plus pricing, and other cost accounting techniques to make decisions

▼ Improving capacity utilization everywhere locally

▼ Holding inventory closer to the customer

▼ A push supply chain

▲ There is a perception that Constraints Management is complex. On the contrary, one of the pillars of Constraints Management is the notion of inherent simplicity. Based on the assumption many scientists hold, that there are no contradictions in nature, Constraints Management solutions strive for clarity and harmony. Often solutions developed using its tools are seen as "obvious" or "commonsense," even for difficult problems to which organizations previously had no solution.

▲ Traditional measurement systems emphasize containing operating expenses rather than expanding throughput.

▲ There is a perception that Constraints Management is relevant only in manufacturing environments. The same was once said of the Toyota Production System and Six Sigma, yet they have been implemented successfully in healthcare.

▲ Constraints Managements can be seen as in competition with Lean and Six Sigma rather than complementary.

▲ Constraints Management uses several management terms in a manner that is not consistent with their traditional meaning.

▲ There is a perception that Constraints Management is time-consuming.

It is true that Constraints Management tools and concepts sometimes require multiple paradigm shifts and radical cultural change. If an organization cannot handle radical changes fast, we recommend introduction of Constraints Management tools slowly, in a gradual manner, into Lean and Six Sigma cultures, similar to "boiling a frog" by increasing the heat slowly. Attempting to force an organization to adopt Constraints Management before it is ready will be met with failure, just like trying to put a frog into a pot of water that is already boiling. Same as the frog would immediately jump out to escape, cultural change in organizations is just as delicate. We recommend a phased approach, where some steps can occur concurrently, as follows:

1. Getting leadership onboard—justification for integrating Constraints Management
2. Active leadership engagement, including both the CEO and the CFO
3. Hands-on training at leadership and practitioner levels
4. Practicing Constraints Management tools and concepts requiring minor change in paradigm and information technology (IT) infrastructure
5. Piloting radically different concepts requiring major paradigm shifts
6. Mentoring practitioners and coaching leadership
7. Measuring the bottom-line difference—quantifying the breakthrough
8. Full-scale implementation of Constraints Management concepts with Lean Six Sigma

Even though we have observed grassroots applications of Constraints Management leading to full deployments later, *obtaining leadership buy-in* first is highly recommended. When enlisting the support of leadership, the following should be communicated:

▲ Emphasize the importance of global rather than local improvements.

▲ Highlight the synergy among Lean, Six Sigma, and Constraints Management—their complementary features and benefits.

▲ Focus on the right problem and the right solution at the right time.

▲ Use appropriate healthcare and situational examples related to Constraints Management.

▲ Take advantage of opportunities to point out the limitations of an incomplete toolset.

▲ Reinforce that the problem and data determine the tools to be used.

▲ Reaffirm that methodology selection is not a matter of choice or dogma.

▲ Use simplified language, and translate jargon terminology to relevant vernacular.

▲ Demonstrate proof of concept with hands-on simulations and exercises.

It is also beneficial to address differences among Constraints Management and Lean when introducing the integrated approach. There are some nuances but nothing that prevents integration. Constraints Management is well suited for systems that experience high variability in process times but also show high variability in service demand, such as hospitals. Known for its robustness against variation, the buffer management approach is a dynamic real-time feedback system that makes potential problems very visible without creating false alarms.

Why should an organization bring yet another methodology, another tool set into their tool box and into their busy lives? Can they achieve major breakthroughs by bringing in Constraints Management with a much higher ROI than with isolated deployments of Lean and/or Six Sigma? There is growing evidence that they can.

The first success stories of the integrated approach emerged from the manufacturing and defense industries. Russ Pirasteh conducted controlled implementations of stand-alone Lean and Six Sigma methods versus an integrated application of Constraints Management with Lean Six Sigma across 21 plants of SCI Sanmina, a global electronics manufacturer. The integrated application resulted in a contribution of 89 percent of the total savings reported. On the other hand, stand-alone Six Sigma and stand-alone Lean deployments provided 7 and 4 percent contribution to company savings, respectively.

Concurrently, we saw the impact of an integrated approach our team applied at the U.S. Naval Aviation Enterprise starting in 2006 with two other core contractors. Our team's mission was to transform the aviation maintenance and supply chain through the application of continuous process-improvement methodologies, specifically integration of theory of constraints and Lean Six Sigma, in order to better support war fighter requirements. In 2008, our team won the award for logistics and industrial operations. Savings exceeded $300 million.

Success stories of the integrated approach started to emerge from healthcare as well. For example, Accugenix, a service laboratory based in Newark, Delaware, used an integrated approach to increase service levels to customers while simultaneously decreasing costs and variability for DNA testing. As a result, laboratory capacity was more than doubled, and overall business capacity increased by 25 percent with no staffing increases, as Michael Pitcher describes in his recent ASQ article, "The Challenge of Overcoming Success." He wrote "Conventional approaches deploy Lean, Six Sigma, or TOC as a single process-improvement method. In this case, creating a process-improvement strategy that employed all three was crucial to achieving sustainable breakthrough performance for Accugenix."

Dr. Gary Wadhwa applied an integrated approach at Adirondack Oral & Maxillofacial Surgery. An integrated approach allowed him to increase his profits from $101,184 in 2001 to $2,517,039 in 2007. This almost 25-fold increase in profits definitely is a breakthrough improvement, as he described at the Theory of Constraints International Certification Organization (TOCICO) 2009 Conference.

Impressive results also have been reported from an integrated application at MD Anderson Cancer Center. In addition to an estimated savings of $2,447,000 over four years, the center consolidated laboratories from four to two. The center reduced inpatient turnaround time by 36 percent, and outpatient fast-track turnaround time was reduced by 17 percent, according to a presentation by Sherry Martin.

These are a few compelling success stories. If executive leadership is convinced about the benefits of Constraints Management, deployment can begin. Next, active leadership engagement is necessary for introducing Constraints Management, similar to Lean and Six Sigma deployments. A highly visible, genuine commitment will accelerate culture change.

Subsequently, we recommend practicing Constraints Management tools and concepts requiring minor change with no software changes required. These include selected thinking processes tools for project selection and reprioritization, as well as conflict resolution. Process-improvement projects, such as Six Sigma and rapid improvement workshops, also benefit from injection of thinking processes tools.

In addition, we recommend incorporating the five focusing steps into process-level value-stream analyses. Selected critical chain project-management principles also can be implemented right away, as described in Chapter 2. Ideally, Throughput decision support should be introduced to the finance department at the very beginning because evaluating the impact will depend on the method used for benefits. However, in practice, finance departments have been quite slow in embracing this approach. Changing the relative importance of Throughput versus operating expenses in the eyes of the CFOs appears to be quite challenging.

Hands-on training and mentoring, particularly practical simulations, are very useful to get buy-in. Many exercises were developed to teach various Constraints Management concepts, which include

- ▲ Dice game
- ▲ Nickel game
- ▲ Dollar game
- ▲ Job-shop game
- ▲ Assembly game
- ▲ Alpha-number-shape game
- ▲ Sixes game
- ▲ Bead game
- ▲ Velocé

When Lean, Six Sigma, and Constraints Management were integrated for the Enterprise AIRSpeed project of Naval Aviation Enterprise, we jointly developed a paper airplane exercise with other core contractor team members. Called *Velocé*, this exercise shows that when these three methodologies are implemented in concert, profits and Throughput increase dramatically, whereas flow times, inventories, operating expenses, and defects decrease significantly. Figure 7.5 shows the bottleneck identified by the participants in the exercise.

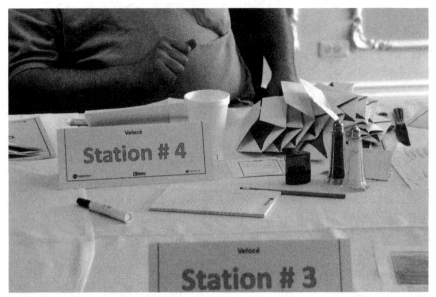

Figure 7-5 Velocé simulation.

After seeing the impact of the Constraints Management tools that are easiest to implement, piloting is recommended for radically different concepts requiring *paradigm shifts*. These include

▲ Drum-buffer-rope/buffer management
▲ Dynamic replenishment
▲ Full-scale implementation of critical chain project management
▲ Throughput decision support

To enable dynamic process management, many of these solutions require availability of specific data updates and specialized software with the IT infrastructure for the retrieval of these data. Many hospitals do not know how much medication is used on a particular day. Without a system in place to track daily consumption and supply, it is not possible to implement the replenishment solution effectively. Similarly, most successful critical chain applications use specialized software to ensure resource leveling (avoiding multitasking) during planning and to track project buffer consumption during project execution management.

Results speak louder than words. Showcasing the results of improvements using Constraints Management solutions is highly recommended. This is what GE Healthcare (then GE Medical Systems) and GE Aircraft Engine Services did when GE, as a corporation, initially resisted adding Lean to Six Sigma. These two businesses quietly incorporated Lean into their highly successful Six Sigma deployments by allowing the problem drive methodology selection and then letting the results speak for themselves. After an initial period of exclusionist denial, GE very quickly incorporated Lean into its Six Sigma toolset. In the data-driven environment of Six Sigma, it is difficult to argue with what all the data are saying. After reaching a level of readiness, full-scale implementation of Constraints Management with Lean and Six Sigma and beyond can commence.

How To Retool Performance-Improvement Programs

One example of a successful adaptation of performance-improvement tools over time is FedEx Corporation. An early adopter of Total Quality Management, FedEx and its family of companies added to the brand have incorporated tools from the Lean, Six Sigma, and other performance-improvement toolsets as the needs of the business have changed. The company has a core culture of process improvement and has not said "Let's do Lean" or "Let's implement Six Sigma." As performance-improvement methodologies have evolved, FedEx has taken the tools that work and incorporated them into its toolbox. Much has been written about the company's success in maintaining a quality culture while growing, changing, innovating, and adapting in a rapidly changing business landscape. From early examples, such as becoming the first service company granted ISO9001 accreditation and winning a Malcolm Baldrige National Quality Award for operational excellence through recent awards for innovation in the area of green business, FedEx has maintained nimble response to change while maintaining its focus on quality processes.

This example illustrates the benefit of having a flexible and robust performance-improvement toolbox coupled with the business intelligence to use the right tools at the right time. The tools that work in one hospital climate may not work in another. It is also evident that a disconnect between an organization's innovators and process improvement can be disastrous in an environment that is changing at today's pace. What can an organization do to close the gap?

One facet of healthcare organizations that sustains performance improvement and innovation through both good times and bad is the commitment to continue investing in improvement—even when business pressures mount. In these organizations, there may be temporary pushes to get more work done with fewer people by working people harder, but over the long term, these organizations continue to resource improving the processes themselves, allowing people to produce more—working *smarter not harder*. These organizations take advantage of the *system dynamics* of process improvement—the feedback loops in the interactions of people, processes, and culture within the organization. System dynamics is an approach to understanding the behavior of complex systems over time. It deals with internal feedback loops and time delays that affect the behavior of the entire system.

A study by the MIT Center for Innovation in Product Development examined performance-improvement and learning programs in over a dozen cases of the dynamics of implementation and organizational change. Their research makes a compelling case for why sustainment of process improvement is so difficult for many organizations—not because the tools do not work, not because employees or managers are "bad," but rather because the feedback loops in a business system reinforce behaviors that ultimately are bad for the health of the system. Instead of investing in performance improvement continuously, organizations succumb to behaviors that land them in a cycle of eroding capability over the long term.

Looking again at the success of some of the companies discussed here, we can see that whether consciously recognized through the lens of system dynamics or not, companies that establish a culture where improvements in process and innovations in services and products are encouraged, valued, incented, and rewarded are often the companies that are able to remain agile in the face of mounting pressure.

The focus can be kept on engagement while regularly retooling to meet changing business needs. This requires a disciplined approach to evaluating and reevaluating our needs and strategy. Our integrated approach ensures flexibility, giving an organization the right tools at the right time. In addition, structured deployment review ensures that changes in a business's direction can be incorporated quickly into the process-improvement effort.

Conclusion

Sustaining a deployment is a never-ending activity. New issues, combined with the quest to improve even more—the quest for perfection—results in needing to continually *sharpen the saw*. In addition to successfully improving processes and providing better care, the organization also must eliminate or reduce the dependence on external help.

While some organizations make a business decision to continue to outsource practitioner training, the skills development of internal practitioners must be addressed. The approaches to performance improvement are evolving, just like those applied within the delivery of care. Recognition of this evolution should encourage the leadership to explore the next steps in performance improvement, similar to physicians keeping abreast of new treatments and medicines as part of licensure mandates.

Many performance-improvement deployments tend to plateau—or reach a point where it may seem that no additional improvement can be realized or at least the level of improvements and the return on performance-improvement investment may decrease—the point of diminishing returns. When this starts occurring, the executive leadership team must take action to reenergize the deployment. How this is done is very organization-specific. Most important, the path to sustainment requires organizational commitment over an extended period of time. A performance-improvement deployment without sustainment is like building a house without a foundation—lacking support, it will crumble.

On a final note, it is our hope that this book will enable readers to understand that performance improvement requires systems thinking and an integrated approach. Our intent has been to allow the reader to apply commonsense breakthrough solutions to manage bottlenecks, eliminate waste, reduce errors, and contain costs in healthcare organizations. Improving quality of care and efficiency while effectively managing constraints means that organizations can provide world-class healthcare while remaining financially viable. This is not an either/or; it is about the patient and the money. Without a focus on both, healthcare organizations cannot continue to do what they are in business to do—healing patients. Lean, Six Sigma, and Constraints Management impel us to strive for perfection. The race to perfection has no finish line. Performance improvement itself is not exempt from continuous improvement. There is always a better solution just beyond the horizon and a way out of the bottleneck.

APPENDIX

Reliability and Validity of Assessment Measures

A great deal of effort was expended to ensure both the reliability and validity of these assessments. Internal consistency was used as the approach in measuring reliability. Each assessment was meant to be administered multiple times to skilled practitioners to rate organizations with which they had been associated. During each assessment's development, the internal consistency of each construct was measured using Cronbach's coefficient alpha, which is the most common statistic used to quantify the degree to which all items within a given construct measure the same attribute. Based on a review of scholarly literature, a minimum alpha level of 0.7 was applied. Only items that were included in the final alpha calculation are included in the instrument. The range across all constructs of the performance improvement maturity assessment was between 0.8147 and 0.9085. The range across all constructs for the change-readiness assessment was between 0.8212 and 0.9085

To assess face validity, each instrument was reviewed by several subject matter experts (SMEs) to ensure the understandability of all items. For construct validity, a separate set of trained performance-improvement practitioners reviewed the instruments and felt that each item really measured what it was intended to measure. Concurrent validity was difficult to determine because most other maturity models are simply descriptive in nature and do not include an assessment instrument. Concurrent validity also was challenging to determine for the change-readiness assessment because its results could not be compared with those of other instruments within the same organization. During the test for internal consistency, the overall findings were compared with the practitioner estimate of the respective organization's maturity and change-readiness levels. The alignment of these expert estimates with the results of the instrument was used to confirm concurrent validity, as prescribed by Litwin. Assessing the predictive validity of each assessment is an ongoing activity that we hope this book's readers will contribute to by providing the results of any use of these instruments along with comments on efficacy relating to predicting the current maturity state and change-readiness level of the organization. Please provide your results (feel free to mask any organizational information as you deem appropriate) to bookfeedback@novaces.com.

Performance-Improvement Maturity Assessment

All items in this survey will be assessed using a five-item scale ranging from "Strongly Disagree" to "Strongly Agree."

1. My organization has a structured approach for solving complex quality-related problems.
   - ❏ Strongly Disagree
   - ❏ Disagree
   - ❏ Neutral
   - ❏ Agree
   - ❏ Strongly Agree

2. Within my organization, a plan has been developed that outlines the path forward for deploying continuous process improvement.
   - ❏ Strongly Disagree
   - ❏ Disagree
   - ❏ Neutral
   - ❏ Agree
   - ❏ Strongly Agree

3. Leaders in my organization follow up to ensure that improvements are implemented and applied over time.
   - ❏ Strongly Disagree
   - ❏ Disagree
   - ❏ Neutral
   - ❏ Agree
   - ❏ Strongly Agree

4. My organization actively pursues opportunities to quickly implement obvious and low-risk improvements.
   ❏ Strongly Disagree
   ❏ Disagree
   ❏ Neutral
   ❏ Agree
   ❏ Strongly Agree

5. My organization regularly communicates improvement activity successes.
   ❏ Strongly Disagree
   ❏ Disagree
   ❏ Neutral
   ❏ Agree
   ❏ Strongly Agree

6. Action has been taken to examine process-level metrics and plan continuous-process-improvement-specific activities.
   ❏ Strongly Disagree
   ❏ Disagree
   ❏ Neutral
   ❏ Agree
   ❏ Strongly Agree

7. My organization continually assesses our progress in implementing continuous process improvement.
   ❏ Strongly Disagree
   ❏ Disagree
   ❏ Neutral
   ❏ Agree
   ❏ Strongly Agree

8. A formal program is in place to develop highly skilled continuous-process-improvement practitioners through a rigorous apprenticeship or advanced training program.
   ❏ Strongly Disagree
   ❏ Disagree
   ❏ Neutral
   ❏ Agree
   ❏ Strongly Agree

9. My organization has developed a process to identify and select practitioners to be trained in the application of continuous-process-improvement methods.
   - ❏ Strongly Disagree
   - ❏ Disagree
   - ❏ Neutral
   - ❏ Agree
   - ❏ Strongly Agree

10. The change readiness of my organization has been assessed, and specific actions are underway to improve readiness.
    - ❏ Strongly Disagree
    - ❏ Disagree
    - ❏ Neutral
    - ❏ Agree
    - ❏ Strongly Agree

11. My organization has developed highly skilled practitioners who can advise less experienced practitioners as well as leaders in continuous-process-improvement concepts and practices.
    - ❏ Strongly Disagree
    - ❏ Disagree
    - ❏ Neutral
    - ❏ Agree
    - ❏ Strongly Agree

12. Gaps between my organization's strategic goals and performance have been reviewed, and action plans have been developed to mitigate any gaps.
    - ❏ Strongly Disagree
    - ❏ Disagree
    - ❏ Neutral
    - ❏ Agree
    - ❏ Strongly Agree

13. My organization has articulated a specific approach or set of methods to apply within our continuous-process-improvement efforts.
   ❏ Strongly Disagree
   ❏ Disagree
   ❏ Neutral
   ❏ Agree
   ❏ Strongly Agree

14. Core processes have been identified by senior leaders, and actions have been taken to ensure that performance expectations are being met.
   ❏ Strongly Disagree
   ❏ Disagree
   ❏ Neutral
   ❏ Agree
   ❏ Strongly Agree

15. My organization has validated significant benefits from our continuous-process-improvement efforts.
   ❏ Strongly Disagree
   ❏ Disagree
   ❏ Neutral
   ❏ Agree
   ❏ Strongly Agree

16. A plan has been developed outlining specific training required based on position and role within my organization.
   ❏ Strongly Disagree
   ❏ Disagree
   ❏ Neutral
   ❏ Agree
   ❏ Strongly Agree

Change-Readiness Assessment

All items in this survey will be assessed using a five-item scale ranging from "Strongly Disagree" to "Strongly Agree."

1. Decisions are made quickly and close to the problem by those most knowledgeable and affected.
   - ❏ Strongly Disagree
   - ❏ Disagree
   - ❏ Neutral
   - ❏ Agree
   - ❏ Strongly Agree

2. People in my work unit feel personally responsible for the quality of my work.
   - ❏ Strongly Disagree
   - ❏ Disagree
   - ❏ Neutral
   - ❏ Agree
   - ❏ Strongly Agree

3. People in my work unit have good teamwork skills.
   - ❏ Strongly Disagree
   - ❏ Disagree
   - ❏ Neutral
   - ❏ Agree
   - ❏ Strongly Agree

4. People in my work unit have the skills needed to improve the efficiency and effectiveness of our work.
   - ❏ Strongly Disagree
   - ❏ Disagree
   - ❏ Neutral
   - ❏ Agree
   - ❏ Strongly Agree

5. Senior leaders are adept at planning and implementing change.
   - ❑ Strongly Disagree
   - ❑ Disagree
   - ❑ Neutral
   - ❑ Agree
   - ❑ Strongly Agree

6. When appropriate, teams are used in my agency to accomplish goals.
   - ❑ Strongly Disagree
   - ❑ Disagree
   - ❑ Neutral
   - ❑ Agree
   - ❑ Strongly Agree

7. Senior leaders clearly communicated the need for continuously improving the quality of our products/services.
   - ❑ Strongly Disagree
   - ❑ Disagree
   - ❑ Neutral
   - ❑ Agree
   - ❑ Strongly Agree

8. I would trust my immediate work supervisor during a period of significant change.
   - ❑ Strongly Disagree
   - ❑ Disagree
   - ❑ Neutral
   - ❑ Agree
   - ❑ Strongly Agree

9. There are few levels between the individual contributors and the head of the business unit.
   - ❑ Strongly Disagree
   - ❑ Disagree
   - ❑ Neutral
   - ❑ Agree
   - ❑ Strongly Agree

10. People in my work unit do a good job of communicating and exchanging information with other parts of the organization.
    - ❏ Strongly Disagree
    - ❏ Disagree
    - ❏ Neutral
    - ❏ Agree
    - ❏ Strongly Agree

11. People in my work unit help one another solve problems.
    - ❏ Strongly Disagree
    - ❏ Disagree
    - ❏ Neutral
    - ❏ Agree
    - ❏ Strongly Agree

12. People in my work unit have the knowledge and skills needed to operate successfully in the changing environment, and we have a good development pipeline.
    - ❏ Strongly Disagree
    - ❏ Disagree
    - ❏ Neutral
    - ❏ Agree
    - ❏ Strongly Agree

13. People in my agency participate in cross-unit and cross-functional teams to accomplish goals.
    - ❏ Strongly Disagree
    - ❏ Disagree
    - ❏ Neutral
    - ❏ Agree
    - ❏ Strongly Agree

14. People in my work unit are actively involved in improving work processes and services.
    - ❏ Strongly Disagree
    - ❏ Disagree
    - ❏ Neutral
    - ❏ Agree
    - ❏ Strongly Agree

15. People in my work unit believe that they will be able to do what the organization is expecting of them.
- ❏ Strongly Disagree
- ❏ Disagree
- ❏ Neutral
- ❏ Agree
- ❏ Strongly Agree

16. I would trust senior leaders during a period of significant change.
- ❏ Strongly Disagree
- ❏ Disagree
- ❏ Neutral
- ❏ Agree
- ❏ Strongly Agree

17. I know how my job contributes to achieving the overall mission and goals of the organization.
- ❏ Strongly Disagree
- ❏ Disagree
- ❏ Neutral
- ❏ Agree
- ❏ Strongly Agree

18. Senior leaders have a clear vision of the future, and the vision is understood throughout the organization.
- ❏ Strongly Disagree
- ❏ Disagree
- ❏ Neutral
- ❏ Agree
- ❏ Strongly Agree

19. The tasks I accomplish are viewed as important to the success of the organization.
- ❏ Strongly Disagree
- ❏ Disagree
- ❏ Neutral
- ❏ Agree
- ❏ Strongly Agree

20. People in my work unit have the skills needed to perform our current jobs effectively.
❏ Strongly Disagree
❏ Disagree
❏ Neutral
❏ Agree
❏ Strongly Agree

21. I am satisfied with how information is communicated about important changes.
❏ Strongly Disagree
❏ Disagree
❏ Neutral
❏ Agree
❏ Strongly Agree

22. Those most affected are involved in diagnosing the problem and making recommendations.
❏ Strongly Disagree
❏ Disagree
❏ Neutral
❏ Agree
❏ Strongly Agree

23. I know my organization's mission and goals.
❏ Strongly Disagree
❏ Disagree
❏ Neutral
❏ Agree
❏ Strongly Agree

24. I get the information I need to do a good job.
❏ Strongly Disagree
❏ Disagree
❏ Neutral
❏ Agree
❏ Strongly Agree

25. This is an organization that supports risk-taking and change.
❏ Strongly Disagree
❏ Disagree
❏ Neutral
❏ Agree
❏ Strongly Agree

Event Charter

<Insert Event Title> Charter

Event Information						
Event type		ProcessVSA	☐	Rapid improvement workshop		☐
Title:				Charter date:		
Location:						
Metrics:		Unit	Baseline	Entitlement		Target
<Primary metric>						
<Secondary metric >						
Benefiting customer(s):						
Event mission:						
Event start date:		Event completion date:		Project closure date:		
Event Team						
Event champion:				Lead practitioner:		
Finance representative:				Process owner:		
Team members:						
Operational Definition						
<Discuss the operational definitions associated with the metrics addressed above.>						

Problem Statement

Strategic Alignment

<Describe how the event will affect strategic goals that are checked below.>
☐   <Strategic goal 1>
☐   <Strategic goal 2>
☐   <Strategic goal 3>

Business Case

Benefits: <Address how the organization will benefit by successful completion of the event. Address specific financial benefits when possible.>

Financial: ☐	Operational/mission: ☐

Project scope:

  In scope:

  Out of scope:

Process start event:	Process stop event:

Event Authorizations

	Champion signature	Date	Facilitator signature	Date
Event charter				

REFERENCES

Ackoff, Russell. "From Mechanistic to Social Systemic Thinking." *Systems Thinking in Action Conference*. Boston, MA: Pegasus Communications, Inc., 1993.

Adrian, Nicole. "Don't Just Talk the Talk." *Quality Progress*, July 2009, pp. 31–33.

Adunka, Robert. "Teaching TRIZ Within Siemens." *TrizFuture2008 Conference*. Enschede, Netherlands, 2008.

Afinitus Group, LLC. "Public Works in Japan: Leading the Way Again—Japanese Government Embraces Critical Chain." Afinitus.com, November 26–27, 2008; available at: www.afinitus.com/japanpw.html; accessed September 22, 2010.

After Action Review; available at: http://afteractionreview.com/; accessed November 18, 2010.

Alexander, M. "Six Sigma Simplified: Quantum Improvement Made Easy." *Technometrics* 44(2):2003.

American Hospital Association. *Report on the Economic Crisis: Initial Impact on Hospitals*. Chicago: American Hospital Association, 2008.

American Society for Quality. *Certification*. Milwaukee, WI, 2010; available at: http://asq.org/certification/index.html; accessed November 18, 2010.

Amin, Zina. "TRIZ Innovation for Healthcare: A Tool for Generating Breakthrough Improvements." *WCBF Lean Six Sigma and Business Improvement in Healthcare Summit* 2010. New Orleans, LA, 2010.

ANCC Magnet Recognition Program. Silver Spring, MD, 2010; available at: www.nursecredentialing.org/Magnet.aspx; accessed November 8, 2010.

Anonymous. "Black Belts Save Motorola a Billion." *Strategic Direction* 18(1):2002.

Anonymous. "Medicare and Medicaid: Texas Hospital Saves $2.8 Million in One Year with Help from Premier Healthcare Alliance's Performance Improvement Program." *Elder Law Weekly*, August 2010, p. 3279.

Anonymous. "Quality of Care: Electronic Recordkeeping Boosts Patient Safety, Saves DMC More than $5 Million—For Second Straight Year." *Telemedicine Law Weekly*, September 2010.

Antony, Jiju, Alex Douglas, and Frenie Jiju Antony. "Determining the Essential Characteristics of Six Sigma Black Belts." *TQM Magazine* 19(3):2007.

Army Combined Arms Command. "A Leader's Guide to After-Action Reviews." Training Circular 25-20. Washington: Department of the Army, September 30, 1993.

ASQ Lean Six Sigma Hospital Study Advisory Committee. "Get Your Checkup." *Quality Progress*, August 2009, pp. 44–50.

Azzopardi, Sandro. *The Evolution of Project Management*. Available at: www.projectsmart.co.uk/pdf/evolution-of-project-management.pdf; accessed September 22, 2010.

Baldrige by Sector: Health Care. Gaithersburg, MD, October 5, 2010; available at: www.nist.gov/baldrige/enter/health_care.cfm; accessed November 8, 2010.

Batalden, Paul B., and Julie J. Mohr. "An Invitation from Florence Nightingale: Come and Learn About Improving Healthcare." In Joint Commission on Accreditation of Healthcare Organizations, ed., *Florence Nightingale: Measuring Hospital Care Outcomes*. Oakbrook Terrace: Joint Commission on Accreditation of Healthcare Organizations, 1999, pp. 11–15, Washington,

Bemis-Daugherty, Anita, and Mary Fran Delaune. "Reducing Patient Falls in Inpatient Settings." *PT*, May 2008.

Benedetto, A. R. "Adapting Manufacturing-Based Six Sigma Methodology to the Service Environment of a Radiology Film Library." *Journal of Healthcare Management* 48(4):2003.

Bertels, Thomas, ed. *Rath & Strong's Six Sigma Leadership Handbook*. Hoboken, NJ: Wiley, 2003.

Bertels, Thomas, and George Patterson. "Measuring and Auditing Results." In Thomas Bertels, ed., *Six Sigma Leadership Handbook*. Hoboken, NJ: Rath and Strong, 2003, pp. 458–477.

Berwick, Donald M., A. Blanton Godfrey, and Jane Roessner. *Curing Health Care: New Strategies for Quality Improvement*. San Francisco: Jossey-Bass, 2002.

Berwick, Donald M., Thomas W. Nolan, and John Whittington. "The Triple Aim: Care, Health, and Cost." *Health Affairs*, May–June 2008.

Bhote, K. R. *The Ultimate Six Sigma: Beyond Quality Excellence to Total Business Excellence*. New York: AMACOM/American Management Association, 2002.

Birnbaum, David, and Rita L. Radcliffe. "Overzealous Oversight of Healthcare Quality Improvement Projects." *Clinical Governance: An International Journal* 13(4):2008.

Bisognano, Maureen. "Engaging the CFO in Quality." *Healthcare Executive*, September–October 2009, pp. 76–78.

Boaden, Ruth, Gill Harvey, Claire Moxham, and Nathan Proudlove. *Quality Improvement: Theory and Practice in Healthcare*. Coventry, United Kingdom: NHS Institute for Innovation and Improvement, 2008.

Borfitz, Deb. "Lilly: New Operating Model Will Speed Tailored Therapies to Market." *eCliniqua*. March 1, 2010; available at: www.ecliniqua.com/eCliniqua_article.aspx?id=97279; accessed September 22, 2010.

Bouchet, Bruno, Irina Stirbu, and Nilufar Rakhmanova. *An Introduction to the Field of Quality Improvement in Health Care*. Technical Report. United States Agency for International Development, Washington, 2006.

Breen, Anne M., Tracey Burton-Houle, and David C. Aaron. "Applying the Theory of Constraints in Health Care: 1. The Philosophy." *Quality Management in Health Care*, 2002.

Burgess, Nicola. "How Is Lean Being Applied to Health? Classifying Approaches to Lean Implementation in the NHS." Ph.D thesis, Warwick Business School, University of Warwick, England, 2009.

Bycio, Peter, Rick D. Hackett, and Joyce S. Allen. "Further Assessments of Bass's (1985) Conceptualization of Transactional and Transformational Leadership." *Journal of Applied Psychology* 80: 468–478, 1995.

Byrnes, John, and Joe Fifer. "Moving Quality to the Top of the Hospital Agenda." *Healthcare Financial Management*, August 2010, pp. 64–69.

Caldwell, Chip. *The Handbook for Managing Change in Healthcare*. Milwaukee, WI: ASQ Quality Press, 1998.

Carey, R. G., and R. C. Lloyd. *Measuring Quality Improvement in Healthcare: A Guide to Statistical Process Control Applications*. New York: Quality Resources, 1995.

Carmines, Edward G., and Richard A. Zeller. *Reliability and Validity Assessment*. Sage Publications, Thousand Oaks, CA, 1979.

Carter, Robert E., Subhash C. Lonial, and P. S. Raju. "Impact of Quality Management on Hospital Performance: An Empirical Examination." *Quality Management Journal* 17(7):2010.

Centers for Medicare and Medicaid Services. *NHE Fact Sheet*. June 29, 2010; available at: www.cms.gov/NationalHealthExpendData/25_NHE_Fact_Sheet.asp; accessed November 10, 2010.

Cerveny, Janice F. "Managing (Improving) Back Office Healthcare Operations." *TOCICO 2009 North American Regional Conference*. Tacoma, WA: Theory of Constraints International Certification Organization, 2009, pp. 1–35.

Chang, R. Y. *Process Reengineering in Action: A Practical Guide to Achieving Breakthrough Results*. London: Kogan Page, 1996.

Chao, Samantha. "The State of Quality Improvement and Implementation Research: Expert Views." Washington: Institute of Medicine, 2007.

Clark, Don. *After Action Reviews*. July 18, 2010; available at: www.nwlink.com/~donclark/leader/leadaar.html; accessed November 18, 2010.

Cleland, David I., and Lewis R. Ireland. *Project Management: Strategic Design and Implementation*. New York: McGraw-Hill, 2002.

Committee on Quality of Health Care in America, Institute of Medicine. *Crossing the Quality Chasm: A New Health System for the 21st Century*. Consensus Report. Washington: Institute of Medicine, 2001.

Conley, David W. "Effective Organizational Integration of TRIZ." In *TRIZCon2009: TRIZ for Tomorrow's Innovations*. Altshuller Institute for TRIZ Studies, Woodland Hills, CA, 2009.

Cox, James F., III, and John G. Schleier, Jr. *Theory of Constraints Handbook*. NY: McGraw-Hill, 2010.

Crosby, Phillip B. *Quality Is Free: The Art of Making Quality Certain*. New York: McGraw-Hill, 1979.

Crosby, Phillip B. *Quality Is Still Free: Making Quality Certain in Uncertain Times*. New York: McGraw-Hill, 1996.

D'Anci, Alex. "Towards Operational Excellence: Applying TOC in a Global Manufacturing Organization." *TOCICO Conference 2008.* Las Vegas, NV: TOCICO, 2008.

Davis, Karen, Cathy Schoen, and Kristof Stremikis. *Mirror, Mirror on the Wall.* New York: The Commonwealth Fund, 2010.

De Feo, Joseph A., and Zion Bar-El. "Creating Strategic Change More Efficiently with a New Design for Six Sigma Process." *Journal of Change Management* 3(1):2002.

De Smet, Eric. "TOC in Healthcare: National University Hospital Singapore." *TOC World.* Uncasville, CT, 2006.

Deming, W. Edwards. *Out of the Crisis.* Cambridge, MA: Massachusetts Institute of Technology Center for Advanced Engineering Study, 1986.

Deming, W. Edwards. *The New Economics: For Industry, Government, Education,* 2d ed. Cambridge, MA: MIT Press, 1994.

Demory, Erin F., and Henry F. Camp. *The Benefits of Moving from a Push to a Pull System.* Charleston, SC, n.d.

DeParle, Nancy-Ann. *The Affordable Care Act Helps America's Uninsured.* September 16, 2010; available at: www.whitehouse.gov/blog/2010/09/16/affordable-care-act-helps-americas-uninsured; accessed November 10, 2010.

Dettmer, H. William. "Constraint Management." *Goal Systems International.* Port Angeles, WA, 2000; available at: www.goalsys.com/books/documents/ConstraintManagement.pdf; accessed December 1, 2010.

Dettmer, H. William. *Goldratt's Theory of Constraints: A Systems Approach to Continuous Improvement.* Milwaukee, WI: ASQ Quality Press, 1997.

Dettmer, H. William. "Strategy." In James F. Cox, III, and John G. Schleier, Jr., eds., *Theory of Constraints Handbook.* New York: McGraw-Hill, 2010, pp. 551–585.

Dettmer, H. William. *The Logical Thinking Process: A Systems Approach to Complex Problem Solving.* Milwaukee, WI: American Society for Quality, 2007.

Dlugaz, Yosef D. *Value-Based Health Care: Linking Finance and Quality.* San Francisco: Wiley, 2010.

Ean, Khaw Choon. "100 Kids 100 Clouds 100 Days." *TOCICO 2006 Conference.* Miami, FL: Theory of Constraints International Certification Organization, 2006, pp. 1–91.

Edmund, Mark. "Quality Key Ingredient in Healthcare Reform." ASQ Quality Progress Web site, 2010. Available at: www.qualityprogress.com; accessed March 1, 2010.

Encinosa, William E., and Fred J. Hellinger. "The Impact of Medical Errors on Ninety-Day Costs and Outcomes: An Examination of Surgical Patients." *Health Services Research,* December 2008.

Eubanks, Paula. "The CEO Experience: TQM/CQI Eubanks." *Hospitals* 66(11): 24–36, 1991.

Faster Patient Treatment with TOC and Buffer Management [in Dutch]. Available at: www.procesverbeteren.nl/TOC/TOC_ziekenhuizen.php.

Fillipo, Brian, James Palermo, Judith Napier, and Ellen Flynn, "Clarity Group." *Crushing Silos: A Leadership Imperative to Ensuring Healthcare Safety in an Era of Healthcare Reform*. Chicago, IL, 2010; available at: www.claritygrp.com; accessed January 12, 2011.

Flower, Joe. "A Conversation with Kenneth R. Pelletier: Sound body, Sound Mind." *Healthcare Forum* 37(5):1994.

Ford Motor Company. "Applying KM to Improve Quality." *Inside Knowledge*, October 10, 2005; available at: www.ikmagazine.com/xq/asp/sid.0/articleid .A2EF7666-7FE1-4E60-9BA7-6374E367A75F/eTitle.Case_study_Ford/qx/ display.htm; accessed November 18, 2010.

Frabotta, D. "Six Sigma Set for Growth" *Managed Healthcare Executive* 12(10): 2002.

Furnham, Adrian. "Remember to Manage Upward: Five Traits Are Important When Assessing the Personality of the Boss and Maintaining a Good Working Relationship." *Financial Times*, May 14, 2002.

Geber, Beverly. "Can TQM Cure Health Care?" *Training* 29(8): 25–32, 1992.

Gemmill, Gary. "Managing Upward Communication." *Personnel Journal* 49(2): 107–110, 1970.

General Electric. "Change Acceleration Process Training." Fairfield, CT: General Electric Company, 2006.

George, Michael L. *Lean Six Sigma: Combining Six Sigma Quality with Lean Speed*. New York: McGraw-Hill, 2002.

George Washington University and Massachusetts General Hospital. "Health Information Technology in the United States: On the Cusp of Change, 2009." Washington, Robert Wood Johnson Foundation, 2009.

Gershon, M. "A Look at the Past to Predict the Future." *Quality Progress*, July, 1996.

Gilbert, G. R., and A. E. Nelson. *Beyond Participative Management: Toward Total Employee Empowerment for Quality*. New York: Quorum Books, 1991.

Goldratt, Eliyahu M. *It's Not Luck*. Great Barrington, MA: North River Press, 1994.

Goldratt, Eliyahu M. "Introduction to TOC—My Perspective." In James F. Cox, III, and John Schleier, Jr. *Theory of Constraints Handbook*. New York: McGraw-Hill, 2010, pp. 3–9.

Goldratt, Eliyahu M. *Critical Chain*. Great Barrington, MA: North River Press, 1997.

Goldratt, Eliyahu M. "Keynote Address." *TOCICO 2010*. Las Vegas, NV: Theory of Constraints International Certification Organization, 2010.

Goldratt, Eliyahu M. *The Choice*. Great Barrington, MA: North River Press, 2008.

Goldratt, Eliyahu M. *The Haystack Syndrome: Sifting Information Out of the Data Ocean*. Great Barrington, MA: North River Press, 1991.

Goldratt, Eliyahu M., and Avraham Goldratt. *TOC Insights into Distribution and Supply-Chain*. Video, Goldratt's Marketing Group, Hamburg, NY, 2009.

Goldratt, Eliyahu M., and Jeffery Fox. *The Goal: A Process of Ongoing Improvement*. Great Barrington, MA: North River Press, 2004.

Goldratt, Eliyahu M., and Jeffery Fox. *The Goal: Excellence in Manufacturing.* Croton-on-Hudson, NY: North River Press, 1984.

Goldratt-Ashlag, Efrat. "The Layers of Resistance—The Buy-In Process According to TOC." In James F. Cox, III, and John Schleier, Jr., *Theory of Constraints Handbook.* New York: McGraw-Hill, 2010, 571–585.

Graban, Mark. *Lean Hospitals.* New York: Productivity Press, 2009.

Green, Andrew. *An Introduction to Health Planning for Developing Health Systems.* Oxford, England: Oxford University Press, 2007.

Halder, Robert B. "Making the Reality Match the Image." *Managing Service Quality* 4(1):31–34, 1994.

Hammer, J., and Michael Champy. *Reengineering the Corporation: A Manifesto for Business Revolution.* New York: HarperBusiness Essentials, 1993.

Hassan, Mahmud, Howard P. Tuckman, Robert H. Patrick, David S. Kountz, and Jennifer L. Kohn. "Cost of Hospital Acquired Infections." *Hospital Topics,* July–September 2010.

Hermann, Kenneth G. "The Healthcare System: Strategies for Improvement—A Joint Commission Perspective," ASQ Meeting May 21, 2002, Healthcare Division Track, Denver, CO, 2002.

Hoerl, Roger. "So Just What Is a Sigma, and Why Do I Need Six of Them?" *Stats,* Spring 2004.

Hoerl, Ronald D., and Roger W. Snee. *Leading Six Sigma: A Step-by-Step Guide Based on Experience with GE and Other Six Sigma Companies.* Upper Saddle River, NJ: Prentice-Hall, 2003.

Holt, James R., and Lynn H. Boyd. "Theory of Constraints in Complex Organizations." In James F. Cox, III, and John Schleier, Jr., *Theory of Constraints Handbook.* New York: McGraw-Hill, 2010, 983–1013.

Hooke, Rachel, MD. "Managing Upwards: A Guide for the Foundation Year Doctor." *British Journal of Hospital Medicine* 70(6):2009.

Huang, Zhao. "Implementing TRIZ Principles with Reliability Considerations." *TRIZCon2009: TRIZ for Tomorrow's Innovations.* Altshuller Institute for TRIZ Studies, Woodland Hills, CA, 2009.

IBM. *Making Change Work.* Somers, NY: IBM Corporation, 2008.

Inozu, Bahadir, Nick Niccolai, Clifford A. Whitcomb, Brian MacClaren, Ivan Radovic, and David Bourg. "New Horizons for Shipbuilding Process Improvement." *Journal of Ship Production* 22:87–88, 2006.

Institute of Medicine. *Crossing the Quality Chasm: A New Health System for the 21st Century.* Consensus Report. Washington: Institute of Medicine, 2001.

International Institute for Labour Studies. *Lean Production and Beyond: Labour Aspects of a New Production Concept.* Geneva: International Institute for Labour Studies, 1993.

Isidore, Chris. *Unemployment Hits 10.2%.* November 6, 2009; available at: http://money.cnn.com/2009/11/06/news/economy/jobs_october/index.htm; accessed November 13, 2010.

J. P. Morgan Chase. "2002 Annual Report." New York, 2002.

Jainendrukumar, T. D. "The Project/Program Management Office (PMO)." *PM World Today* X(1):2008.

Jasper, Melanie, and Mansour Jumaa. *Effective Healthcare Leadership.* Chichester, England: Wiley, 2008.

Joint Commission on Accreditation of Healthcare Organizations. *Florence Nightingale: Measuring Hospital Care Outcomes.* Oakbrook Terrace, IL: Joint Commission on Accreditation of Healthcare Organizations, 1999.

Juran Institute. *Total Quality Management: A Practical Guide.* Wilton, CT: Juran Institute, 1991.

Juran, Joseph M. *A History of Managing for Quality: The Evolution, Trends, and Future Directions of Managing for Quality.* Milwaukee, WI: Quality Press, 1995.

Juran, Joseph M. *Juran on Quality by Design: The New Steps for Planning Quality into Goods and Services.* New York: Free Press, 1992.

Juran, Joseph M. *Juran's Quality Control Handbook*, 4th ed. Edited by Frank M. Gryna. New York: McGraw-Hill, 1988.

Kaplan, Robert S., and David P. Norton. "Using the Balanced Scorecard as a Strategic Management System." *Harvard Business Review* Jan-Feb:75–85, 1996.

Kelly, Robert. "Facts for Healthcare." *Where Can $700 Billion in Waste be Cut from the U.S. Healthcare System?* October 2009; available at: www.factsforhealth care.com/whitepaper/HealthcareWaste.pdf; accessed November 11 2010.

Kershaw, Russ. "Using TOC to 'Cure' Healthcare Problems." *Accounting Management Quarterly* Spring:1–7, 2000.

Kimar, Maneesh, Jiju Antony, and Byung Rae Cho. "Project Selection and Its Impact on the Successful Deployment of Six Sigma." *Business Process Management* 15(5):669–686, 2009.

Knight, Alex, and Roy Stratton. "Managing Patient Flow Using Time Buffers." *TOCICO 2010 Conference.* Las Vegas, NV: Theory of Constraints International Certification Organization, 2010, pp. 1–40.

Kohls, Kevin. "Combining Lean and TOC." *Constraints Management User Conference.* Constraints Management Group. San Antonio, TX. 2010.

Kotter, John. "Leading Change." *Harvard Business Review* 73(2):1995.

Kotter, John. "Leading Change: Why Transformation Efforts Fail." *Harvard Business Review*, March–April 1995.

Kotter, John. *Leading Change.* Cambridge, MA: Harvard Business School Press, 1996.

Kowalski, Jamie C. "Needed: A Strategic Approach to Supply Chain Management." *Healthcare Financial Management* June:90–98, 2009.

Kroch, Eugene Vaughn, Thomas PhD, Koepke, Mark JD, MHA, Roman, Sheila MD, Foster, David PhD, Sinha, Sunil MD, MBA, Levey, Samuel PhD, SM "Hospital Boards and Quality Dashboards." *Patient Safety* 2(1):10–19, 2006.

Langabeer, J. *Health Care Operations Management: A Quantitative Approach to Business and Logistics.* Boston: Jones and Bartlett, 2008.

Lean Enterprise Institute. *What Is Lean?* 2009; available at: www.lean.org/WhatsLean/Principles.cfm; accessed November 10, 2010.

Lechleiter, John C. "Reinventing Invention: Fixing the Engine of Biopharmaceutical Innovation." Speech, Eli Lilly & Co., San Diego, CA, 2009.

LeTourneau, Barbara. "Managing Physician Resistance to Change." *Journal of Healthcare Management*, September 2004.

Levine, Mark. "St. Vincent's Is the Lehman Brothers of Hospitals." *New York Magazine*, October 17, 2010, pp. 24–31, 96–97.

Liker, Jeffrey, and David Meier. *The Toyota Way Fieldbook.* New York: McGraw-Hill, 2006.

Litwin, Mark S. *How to Assess and Interpret Survey Psychometrics*, Vol. 2. Newbury Park, CA: Sage Publications, 2002.

Mabin, Victoria J., and John Davies. "The TOC Thinking Processes: Their Nature and Use—Reflections and Consolidation." In James F. Cox, III, and John Schleier, Jr., *Theory of Constraints Handbook.* New York: McGraw-Hill, 2010, pp. 631–669.

Martin, Sherry. "Moving Patients Across a System of Care 'Better, Faster, Cheaper.'" The University of Texas, M. D. Anderson Cancer Center. Institute for Healthcare Excellence.

McWhirter, D. A. *Managing People: Creating the Team-Based Organization.* Holbrook, MA: Adams Publishing, 1995.

Millhiser, William P., and Joseph G. Szmerekovsky. "Teaching Critical Chain Project Management: An Academic Debate, Open Research Questions, Numerical Examples and Counterarguments." *INFORMS National Meeting.* Institute for Operations Research and the Management Sciences. Washington, 2009, pp. 1–25.

Miner, John B. *Organizational Behavior 1: Essential Theories of Motivation and Leadership.* Armonk, NY: M. E. Sharpe, Inc., 2006.

Motwani, Jaideep, Donald Klein, and Raanan Harowitz. "The Theory of Constraints in Services: 2. Examples from Health Care." *Managing Service Quality* 6(2): 30–34, 1996.

Nave, Dave. "How to Compare Six Sigma, Lean and the Theory of Constraints." *Quality Progress*, March 2002.

Nelson, E. C. "Improving Healthcare Part 1L the Clinical Balanced Scorecard." *Journal of Community and Quality Improvement* 22:243–258, 1996.

Neuhauser, Duncan. "Florence Nightingale: A Passionate Statistician." In Joint Commission on Accreditation of Healthcare Organizations, ed., *Florence Nightingale: Measuring Hospital Care Outcomes.* Oakbrook Terrace, IL: Joint Commission on Accreditation of Healthcare Organizations, 1999, pp. 1–9.

NHS Executive. *Action on Cataracts: Good Practice Guide.* London, January 2000.

Nightingale, Florence. *Notes on Matters Affecting the Health, Efficiency and Hospital Administration of the British Army.* London: Harrison and Sons, 1858.

Nolan, Thomas, and Maureen Bisognano. "Finding the Balance Between Quality and Cost." *Healthcare Financial Management* 60(4):1–6, 2006.

Noreen, Eric W., Debra A. Smith, and James T. MacKey. *Theory of Constraints and Its Implications for Management Accounting*. Great Barrington, MA: North River Press, 1995.

Norton, William I., and Lyle Sussman. "Team Charters: Theoretical Foundations and Practical Implications for Quality and Performance." *Quality Management Jounal* 16(1):2009.

O'Conor, Darren. *Business Planning*. Broadstairs, United Kingdom: Scitech Educational, 2000.

Olson, Diane J. "A Study of the Relationships in Financial Performance, Organization Size, Business Classification, and Program Maturity of Six Sigma Systems." Indiana State University, Terre Haute, IN. September 22, 2010.

Page, Rick. *Hope Is Not a Strategy: The 6 Keys to Winning the Complex Sale*. New York: McGraw-Hill, 2003.

Pande, Peter S., Robert P. Neuman, and Roland R. Cavanaugh. *The Six Sigma Way Team Fieldbook: An Implementation Guide for Process Improvement*. New York: McGraw-Hill, 2002.

Peregrim, Drew. *Use Point System for Better Six Sigma Project Selection*. Available at: http://isixsigma.com/index.php?option=com_k2&view=item&id=1144&Itemid=1&Itemid=1; accessed November 11, 2010.

Pexton, Carolyn. "Communication Strategies for Six Sigma Initiatives." *iSixSigma*; available at: http://isixsigma.com/index.php?option=com_k2&view=item&id=677&Itemid=1&Itemid=1; accessed October 28, 2010.

Pexton, Carolyn. "Overcoming Organizational Barriers to Change in Healthcare." *Financial Times*, February 23, 2009, pp. 1–3.

Phipps, Belinda. "Hitting the Bottleneck." *Health Management*, (2) 1999.

Pirasteh, R. M., and Robert E. Fox. *Profitability with No Boundaries: Focus, Reduce Waste, Contain Variability, Optimize TOC, Lean, and Six Sigma*. Milwaukee, WI: ASQ Quality Press, 2010.

Pittman, Paul H. "Project Management: A More Effective Methodology for the Planning and Control of Projects." Ph.D. dissertation, University of Georgia, Athens, GA. 1994.

Plsek, P. E. "Evidence-Based Quality Improvement, Principles, and Perspecitves." *Pediatrics* 103(1):1999.

Plummer, Daryl, and Elise Olding. *Gartner's Interview with Dr. Geary Rummler*. 2010; available at: www.gartner.com/research/fellows/asset_215649_1176.jsp; accessed November 12, 2010.

Porter, Michael E. *Redefining Health Care*. Boston: Harvard Business School Press, 2006.

Project Management Institute. *A Guide to the Project Management Body of Knowledge*, Vol. 3. Newtown Square, PA: Project Management Institute, 2004.

Project Replication Software Solution. 2006; available at: https://ssl110.alentus.com/sigmaflow/solutions/project_replication.html; accessed November 18, 2010.

Pyzdek, Thomas. "Six Sigma and Beyond." *Quality Digest*, October 2000; available at: www.qualitydigest.com/Oct00/html/sixsigma.html; accessed October 25, 2010.

Reid, Richard A., and Thomas E. Shoemaker. "Using the Theory of Constraints to Focus Operational Improvement Efforts: 1. Defining the Problem." *American Water Works Association Journal* 98(7):63–75, 2006.

Reid, Sally. "Focusing on Ophthalmology Waiting Lists. Using the 'Theory of Constraints' Methodology to Improve Services to Patients." *ImpAct*. NHS Learning Network, March 2000.

Revere, L., and K. K. Black. "Integrating Six Sigma with Total Quality Management: A Case Example for Measuring Medication Errors." *Journal of Healthcare Management* 48(6):377–391, 2003.

Ricketts, John A. "Theory of Constraints in Professional, Scientific, and Technical Services." In James F. Cox, III, and John Schleier, Jr., eds., *Theory of Constraints Handbook*. New York: McGraw-Hill, 2010, pp. 859–878.

Ricketts, John A. *Reaching the Goal: How Managers Improve a Services Business Using Goldratt's Theory of Constraints*. IBM Press, Westford, MA, 2007.

Roberts, Herbert. "TRIZ at General Electric: Edison, Altshuller, and Imagination at Work." *TRIZCon2009: TRIZ for Tomorrow's Innovations*. Altshuller Institute for TRIZ Studies, Woodland Hills, CA, 2009.

Robinson, R. D. *The Empowerment Cookbook: Action Plans for Creating, Sustaining, or Refocusing Empowered Work Teams*. New York: McGraw-Hill, 1997.

Roble, Richard S. "Is Your Organization Spooked by Ghostly Team Performances?" *Quality Progress*, May 1997.

Rogers, Everett M. *Diffusion of Innovations*, 5th ed. New York: Free Press, 2003.

Ronen, Boaz, and Shimeon Pass. "The Revised Focusing Steps of TOC: A Value Creation Approach." *TOCICO 2010 Conference*. Las Vegas, NV: Theory of Constraints International Certification Organization, 2010, pp. 1–48.

Ronen, Boaz, Joseph S. Pliskin, and Shimeon Pass. *Focused Operations Management for Health Services Organizations*. San Francisco: Jossey-Bass, 2006.

Rother, John, and Risa Lavizzo-Mourey. "Addressing the Nursing Workforce: A Critical Element for Healthcare Reform." *Health Affairs* 28(3):620–624, 2009.

Ruth, Boaden, Harvey Gill, Moxham Claire Moxham, and ProudloveNathan Proudlove. "Quality Improvement: Theory and Practice in Healthcare." NHS Institute for Innovation and Improvement, Coventry, United Kingdom, 2008.

Savary, Louis M., and Clare Crawford-Mason. *The Nun and the Bureaucrat: How They Found an Unlikely Cure for America's Sick Hospitals*. CC-M Productions, Inc., Washington, 2006.

Scholtes, Peter R., and Brian L. Joiner. *The Team Handbook*, 3d ed. Madison, WI: Oriel, Inc., 2003.

Schutt, Judith A. "Balancing the Health Care Scorecard." Managed Care, September 2003.

Senge, Peter. *Leading Change*. Cambridge, MA: Harvard Business School Press, 1996.

Senge, Peter M., Art Kleiner, Charlotte Roberts, George Roth, Rick Ross, and Bryan Smith. *The Dance of Change: The Challenges to Sustaining Momentum in Learning Organizations*. New York: Doubleday, 1999.

Shewhart, Walter A., and W. Edwards Deming. *Statistical Method from the Viewpoint of Quality Control*. Washington: U.S. Department of Agriculture Graduate School, 1939.

Shoemaker, Tom, and Richard A. Reid. "Quantifying Throughput in Public Sector Organizations." *TOCICO 2010 Conference*. Las Vegas, NV: Theory of Constraints International Certification Organization, 2010, pp. 1–77.

Sibbald, William, and Thomas Massaro. *The Business of Critical Care: A Textbook for Clinicians Who Manage Special Care Units*. Armonk, NY: Futura Publishing, 1996.

Smith, Debra. *The Measurement Nightmare: How the Theory of Constraints Can Resolve Conflicting Strategies, Policies and Measures*. Boca Raton, FL: St. Lucie Press, 2000.

Smith, Debra, and Jeff Herman. "Resolving Measurement/Performance Dilemmas." In James F. Cox, III, and John Schleier, Jr., eds., *Theory of Constraints Handbook*. New York: McGraw-Hill, 2010, pp. 373–401.

Smits, P. "Using Critical Chain Project Management to Drive Innovation in a General Hospital." *TOCICO 2009 Conference*. Amsterdam, the Netherlands: Theory of Constraints International Certification Organization, 2009.

Smits, Paul. "Using Critical Chain Project Management to Drive Innovation in a General Hospital." *TOCICO 2009 Conference*. Amsterdam, the Netherlands: Theory of Constraints International Certification Organization, 2009, pp. 1–26.

Snee, Ronald D. "Dealing with the Achilles' Heel of Six Sigma Initiatives." *Quality Progress* 34(3):66–72, 2001.

Society of Manufacturing Engineer. *Lean Certification*. 2010; available at: www.sme.org/cgi-bin/certhtml.pl?/cert/lean_certification.htm&&SME&; accessed November 18, 2010.

Spradley, B. W. "Managing Change Creatively." *Journal of Nursing Administration* May :32–37, 1980.

Sproull, Bob. *The Ultimate Improvement Cycle: Maximizing Profits Through the Integration of Lean, Six Sigma, and the Theory of Constraints*. Boca Raton, FL: CRC Press, 2009.

Srinivasan, Mandyam, Darren Jones, and Alex Miller. "Applying Theory of Constraints Principles and Lean Thinking at the Marine Corps Maintenance Center." *Defense Acquisition Review Journal*, August-November, 134–145. Washington, 2004.

Stratton, Roy, and Alex Knight. "Managing Patient Flow Using Time Buffers." *Journal of Manufacturing Technology Management* 21(4):484–498, 2010.

Sullivan, Timothy T., Richard A. Reid, and Brad Cartier. *The Theory of Constraints International Certification Organization Dictionary*. TOCICO, Washington: 2007.

Sweeney, Evan. "Means of Egress" *Remains a Top Joint Commission Citation*. August 20, 2010; available at: http://blogs.hcpro.com/hospitalsafety/2010/08/means-of-egress-remains-as-a-top-joint-commission-citations/; accessed November 17, 2010.

Tague, Nancy R. *The Quality Toolbox*, Vol. 2. Milwaukee, WI: ASQ Quality Press, 2005.

Tapping, D., T. Luster, and T. Shuker. *Value Stream Management: Eight Steps to Planning, Mapping, and Sustaining Lean Improvement*. New York: Productivity Press, 2002.

Taylor, Lloyd J., III, and Don Sheffield. "Goldratt's Thinking Process Applied to Medical Claims Processing." *Hospital Topics* 80:13–21, 2002.

Tellier, Mark R. *DMAIC Project Selection Using a Systematic Approach*. Available at: http://isixsigma.com/index.php?option=com_k2&view=item&id=1077&Itemid=1&Itemid=1; accessed November 11, 2010.

Theory of Constraints International Certification Organization. *Purpose and Vision for the Certification Process*. 2010; available at: www.tocico.org/?page=Certification; accessed November 18, 2010.

Ulrich, Dave, Steve Kerr, and Ron Ashkenas. *The GE Work-Out: How to Implement GE's Revolutionary Method for Busting Bureaucracy and Attacking Organizational Problems—Fast!* New York: McGraw-Hill, 2002.

Umble, Michael, and Elisabeth J. Umble. "Utilizing Buffer Management to Improve Performance in a Healthcare Environment." *European Journal of Operational Research* 174(2):1060–1075, 2006.

Unzicker, D. "The Psychology of Being Put on Hold: An Exploratory Study of Service Quality." *Psychology & Marketing* 16(4):1999.

U.S. Army "Change Management." Office of Business Transformation. November 2010. Available at: www.armyobt.army.mil/cpi-kc-cpi-enablers-change-management.html; accessed November 23, 2010.

Veral, Emre, and Harry Rosen. "Can a Focus on Costs Increase Costs?" *Hospital Materiel Management Quarterly* 22(3):28–35, 2001.

Vitalo, Raphael L., Frank Butz, and Joseph P. Vitalo. *Kaizen Desk Reference Standard*. Hope, ME: Lowrey Press, Singapore, 2003.

Wadwa, Gary. "Viable Vision for Health Care Systems." In James F. Cox, III, and John Schleier, Jr., eds., *Theory of Constraints Handbook*. New York: McGraw-Hill, 2010, pp. 899–953.

Walker, Ed. "The Problems with Project Management." In James F. Cox, III, and John Schleier, Jr., eds., *Theory of Constraints Handbook*. New York: McGraw-Hill, 2010, pp. 13–44.

Wall, J. K. "Lilly Revises Playbook in Effort to Score More 'Touchdowns.'" IBJ.com, September 19, 2009; available at: www.ibj.com/lilly-revises-playbook-in-effort-to-score-more-touchdowns/PARAMS/article/7146; accessed September 22, 2010.

Watson, Kevin J. "A Comparison of DRP and TOC Customer Service Performance Within a Multi-Product, Multi-Echelon Physical Distribution Environment." In *Proceedings of the 33rd Annual Meeting of the Decision Sciences Institute*. San Diego: E-Business Track, 2002, pp. 23–26.

Watson, Kevin J. "Executive Summary: The Theory of Constraints." 2010.

Watson, Kevin J., John H. Blackston, and Stanley C. Gardiner. "The Evolution of a Management Philosophy: The Theory of Constraints." *Journal of Operations Management* 25(2):387–402, 2007.

Weed, Julie. "Factory Efficiency Comes to the Hospital." *New York Times*, July 9, 2010.

Weiner, Bryan J., Halle Amick, and Daniel Lee Shoou-Yih. *Conceptualization and Measurement of Organizational Readiness for Change: A Review of the Literature in Health Services Research and Other Fields*. Medical Care Research and Review, Sage Publications. 2008, 65(4) pp. 379–436. Thousand Oaks, CA.

Weinstein, J. S. "IEs Need to Learn That Making Less of IE Can Make More of It." *Industrial Engineering* 24(12):1992.

Werner, Mark. "From System to Clinic." *Modern Physician* 10(8):10–12, 2006.

Weyant, Daniel J. "Critical Black Belt Mentor Attributes and Self-Efficacy." Ph.D dissertation, Capella University, Minneapolis, MN. June 2009.

Whitlock, Joy. "Theory of Constraints and Buffer Management: Cardiff & Vale NHS Trust." QFI Consulting, December 2006; available at: www.qficonsulting.com/media/documents/Cardiff–Vale-NHS-Trust-hg.pdf; accessed November 17, 2010.

Whole System Measures. Boston: Institute for Healthcare Improvement, 2007.

Wilkinson, Nancy L., and John W. Moran. "Team Charter." *The TQM Magazine*, 10(5)1998.

Wolf, Richard. "Number of Uninsured Americans Rises to 50.7 Million." *USA Today*, September 16, 2010; available at: www.usatoday.com/news/nation/2010-09-17-uninsured17_ST_N.htm; accessed November 17, 2010.

Wolper, Lawrance F., ed. *Physician Practice Management: Essential Operational and Financial Knowledge*. Sudbury, MA: Jones and Bartlett, 2005.

Womack, David E., and Steve Flowers. "Improving System Performance: A Case Study in the Application of the Theory of Constraints." *Journal of Healthcare Management* 44(5):397–497, 1999.

Womack, James P., and Daniel T. Jones. *Lean Thinking: Banish Waste and Create Wealth in Your Corporation*. New York: Free Press, 2003.

Womack, James P., Daniel T. Jones, and Daniel Roos. *The Machine That Changed the World*. New York: Free Press, 1990.

Wright, Julie. "TOC for Large-Scale Healthcare Systems." In James F. Cox, III, and John Schleier, Jr., eds., *Theory of Constraints Handbook*. New York: McGraw-Hill, 2010, pp. 955–979.

Young, Terry, Sally Brailsford, Con Connell, Paul Harper, and Jonathan H Klein. "Using Industrial Processes to Improve Patient Care." *BMJ*, January 2004.

Youngman, Kelvyn. *Caring About Healthcare.* Available at: www.dbrmfg.co.nz/. Accessed November 17, 2010.

Zander, K., and M. Hill. " DataMap: A Dashboard to Guide the Executive Team." *Center for Case Management* 16(1):2001.

Zeithaml, Valarie A., A. Parasuraman, and Leonard L. Berry. *Delivering Quality Service.* New York: Free Press, 1990.

Zephro, Chris. "Integrating the TOC Thinking Process and Six Sigma at Seagate Technologies." *TOCICO 2004 Conference.* Miami, FL: Theory of Constraints Internatonal Certification Organization, 2004.

Zilm, Frank. "Designing for Emergencies: Integrating Operations and Adverse-Event Planning." *Health Facilities Management* 23(11):39–42, 2010.

Zinkgraf, Stephen A. *Six Sigma: The First 90 Days.* Upper Saddle River, NJ: Prentice-Hall, 2006.

INDEX

Italic page numbers reference figures.